"A diagnosis of glioblastoma dramatically impacts a patient and their family, and many treatment decisions need to be made in a short period of time. Dr. Gruber is an expert neurosurgeon and he provides patients and families an invaluable roadmap to help them understand and face the challenges of a malignant brain tumor. I highly recommend this book and will be providing it to my patients and their families."

—Andrew Fabiano, MD, FAANS
Contributing Author, National Standards of Care for Brain Cancer
Professor of Neurosurgery and Oncology
Buffalo, NY

"As a senior executive, I interacted often with neurosurgeon Tom Gruber in executive-level meetings and budget discussions to plan for future needs. It never occurred to me that I would become one of his patients in 2015 when I was diagnosed with a brain tumor and underwent brain surgery. Dr. Gruber has carefully explored ways to help us all by developing this brilliant approach to guide patients and their families from diagnosis through every stage of the journey."

—Bonnie Schrock, MBA, FACHE
Brain Tumor Patient
Former COO, Baptist Health Paducah

"To hear that I had brain cancer was like a sucker punch to the stomach. The words *brain cancer* echoed through my head. Unfortunately, in the meantime, I did the one thing no one should do: research your diagnosis on the internet. No two people are alike; your case will never be the same as anyone else's. This is your story and only your story to write. His book, *Navigating Glioblastoma and High Grade Glioma*, is superbly written in that it provides resourceful and practical advice on how to navigate through this journey with an easy-to-read and easy-to-understand guide not only for the patient, but the family as well."

—Candice Cole
Brain Tumor Patient

"This book is amazing. I can honestly say that so many of the things written about, in layman's terms, are exactly the things that I have heard asked by patients and explained by the nurses. This is such a scary and anxious time for the patient and caregiver who have so many questions—and when they get home and start trying to remember, they realize they did not absorb everything that the doctor told them. Having the information in this easy to read and understand book would be wonderful to provide to each patient with this diagnosis."

—Kimberly Sweeney, RN, MBA
Executive Director, Concierge Services
NCI-Designated Comprehensive Cancer Center in New York State

NAVIGATING
GLIOBLASTOMA
AND HIGH GRADE GLIOMA

DR. THOMAS GRUBER • MARCIA GRUBER-PAGE RN

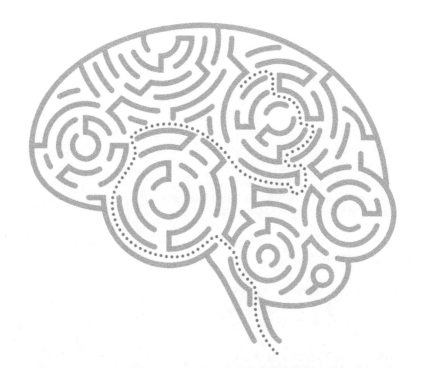

NAVIGATING
GLIOBLASTOMA
AND HIGH GRADE GLIOMA

A patient and family guide to primary brain tumors

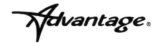

Published by Advantage, Charleston, South Carolina.
Member of Advantage Media Group.

ADVANTAGE is a registered trademark, and the Advantage colophon is a trademark of Advantage Media Group, Inc.

Printed in the United States of America.

10 9 8 7 6 5 4 3 2 1

ISBN: 978-1-64225-409-9 (Paperback)
ISBN: 978-1-64225-426-6 (eBook)

LCCN: 2022912181

Cover design by Analisa Smith.
Layout design by Wesley Strickland.

This publication is designed to provide accurate and authoritative information in regard to the subject matter covered. It is sold with the understanding that the publisher is not engaged in rendering legal, accounting, or other professional services. If legal advice or other expert assistance is required, the services of a competent professional person should be sought.

Advantage Media Group is a publisher of business, self-improvement, and professional development books and online learning. We help entrepreneurs, business leaders, and professionals share their Stories, Passion, and Knowledge to help others Learn & Grow. Do you have a manuscript or book idea that you would like us to consider for publishing? Please visit **advantagefamily.com**.

To Aimee, Caroline, and Meghan for your love, patience, and support in this project. To our patients and their loved ones, hopefully this book will bring them some measure of knowledge, comfort, and control.

ABOUT THIS BOOK

Glioblastoma. The word is intimidating, scary, and confusing, and it will instantly make you feel helpless. Multiple doctors' appointments, strange medical terms, difficult decisions, confusing terminology, and perplexing technology all combine to frighten you and make you wonder how you'll ever navigate this impossible new world and still feel like you're doing everything possible for your own health, or the health of your loved one. This book is designed to clear the fog around glioblastoma and high-grade glioma. To help you as the patient and your loved ones understand the diagnosis in plain, comfortable language. To help you understand the pluses and minuses of the treatment options. To help you make sense of all the testing. To help you understand what to expect at important junctions during treatment. To give you the information you need to make crucial decisions about your care. In this book, I use my fifteen-plus years of knowledge, experience, and training as a board-certified neurosurgeon to guide and shepherd patients diagnosed with glioblastoma and high-grade glioma and their loved ones through this difficult diagnosis.

Some of the questions you might ask could include the following:

- What chemotherapy options are available, and what are the differences?

- Is surgery a good option? Why or why not?

- What is proton beam therapy, and will it help?

I will answer these and many more important questions in a way that will enable you to be confident in your decisions, knowing that you understand all of the options and information coming from your treatment team. In this way you will be able to feel satisfied that you or your loved one is getting the best care available.

CONTENTS

· ·

ABOUT THIS BOOK ix

ACKNOWLEDGMENTS xiii

PREFACE xv

INTRODUCTION 1

CHAPTER 1 5

WHAT IS GLIOBLASTOMA MULTIFORME? IT IS A BEAST ...

CHAPTER 2 13

YOUR TEAM

CHAPTER 3 25

IMAGING TESTS

CHAPTER 4 35

THE COOKBOOK

CHAPTER 5 41

SURGERY

CHAPTER 6 55

CHEMOTHERAPY AND OTHER MEDICATIONS

CHAPTER 7 65

RADIATION THERAPY

CHAPTER 8 71

**NEUROLOGIC DISABILITIES
AND COPING WITH THEM**

CHAPTER 9 81

RECURRENCE

CHAPTER 10 91

ADDITIONAL TREATMENTS

CHAPTER 11 99

**ALTERNATIVE TREATMENTS AND THE ROLE
OF DIET, SUPPLEMENTS, AND ATTITUDE**

CHAPTER 12 111

FINANCIAL CONSIDERATIONS OF GBM

CHAPTER 13 119

OTHER CARE PATHS TO PURSUE OR CONSIDER

CONCLUDING THOUGHTS 129

ABOUT THE AUTHORS 133

CONTACT US 137

ACKNOWLEDGMENTS

I would like to acknowledge the help of Adrienne Jackson, without whom nothing in my life would be done properly or on time. I could never express how much your wonderful attitude, tireless work means to all of our projects.

Suzanna de Boer, your knowledge, talent, experience, and encouragement were invaluable turning this rough idea into a readable, useful tool for patients and families.

Kim Sweeney, Roswell Park Cancer Center, thank you for your guidance and assistance regarding patient and family financial counseling.

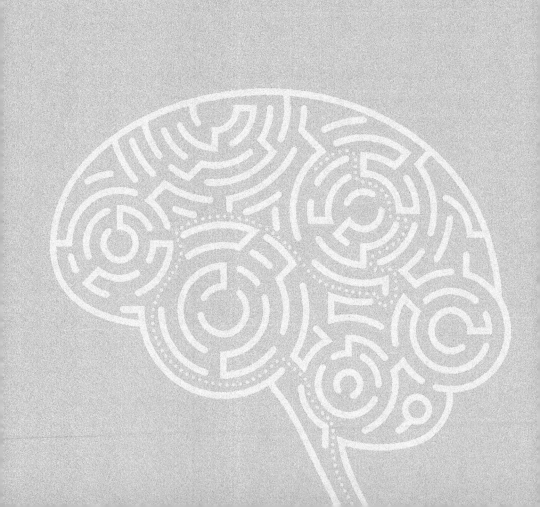

PREFACE

I have been a neurosurgeon for over fifteen years. During that time, I have had approximately thirty thousand patient encounters in the clinic, hospital, and operating room, caring for a variety of neurologic conditions including trauma to the head and spine, Parkinson's disease and movement disorders, congenital and developmental diseases in children, chronic pain conditions, and complicated degenerative conditions of the spine. But it's the work my team and I do with tumors of the brain and spine that is the most challenging and most rewarding.

Patients who have been diagnosed with a tumor of the brain or spine, whether that tumor is benign or cancerous, are terrified that this will shorten their life at worst or result in some sort of disability that will rob them of the life they have imagined and visualized for themselves. These patients and their families require all of our resources to guide them through this diagnosis. Our brain tumor treatment team must provide the most up-to-date medical care, treatment, and counsel, but we also have to be prepared to guide and help our patients and their families through the emotional, practical, spiritual, and financial maze that comes with the life-changing and life-challenging news that you have a brain tumor.

During my career, I have trained, worked, and conducted research alongside some of the best minds in neurosurgery, neuro-oncology, and cancer. First in New York at the University of Buffalo's Jacobs School of Medicine and Biomedical Sciences and at Roswell Park Cancer Center, then joining Baptist Health System in Kentucky, where I have had the pleasure to help plan, develop, and build a brain tumor program from the ground up at the Ray and Kay Eckstein Regional Cancer Care Center.

At Baptist Health in western Kentucky, I have the privilege of working with a team of cancer specialists at the Eckstein cancer center to provide the most up-to-date treatments available for all tumors and cancer diagnoses affecting the brain, spine, and nervous system. We have dedicated our lives and careers to building a program that provides the most cutting-edge technology, expertise, and services that are necessary to provide world-class care of brain tumors for our patients and their families.

INTRODUCTION

Kevin had been diagnosed with brain cancer about two years ago and was returning to our clinic with his family for a routine checkup. I was in my office waiting for them to arrive and pulled up his latest MRI, which had just been done a few minutes earlier. I could immediately see that I was looking at the third recurrence of Kevin's tumor since we initially operated.

I knew his wife Julie always meant business. She showed up to every office visit in a different colorful T-shirt declaring support for brain cancer awareness. She worked desperately to understand her husband's cancer and to support him in every way. I knew the next sixty minutes would be filled with challenging questions: "Where is the recurrence? What does this mean for his overall survival? What are our next options? Do we need to look at experimental trials? Is now the time to return to the University of Arizona to get their opinion?"

Julie and Kevin were thirty-nine and forty years old, respectively, and they had been married for about nine years and had two children aged five and seven when Kevin had a seizure at home. Kevin was a big, solid man standing six foot two, and he worked as a welder. Of course, he had only ever been to the hospital for minor bumps and bruises and had never taken a day off work in his life. His wife, Julie, split her time between taking care of the children and family and working as a teaching assistant.

Kevin was brought to the emergency room, where a CT scan of his brain showed a fuzzy abnormal area in the left front of his brain. In order to get a better idea of what was going on in Kevin's brain and to figure out why he suddenly had a seizure, an MRI with contrast was ordered.

The MRI clearly showed the reason for Kevin's seizure: a well-defined "ring enhancing" mass in the left side of his brain toward the front. This was almost certainly some sort of tumor.

Despite multiple surgeries, chemotherapy, and radiation, Kevin passed away of a brain cancer called glioblastoma multiforme (GBM) about thirty months later. This book is written for Julie, patients with a GBM or high-grade glioma (HGG) diagnosis, and also for all the friends and family that help GBM and HGG patients navigate through this difficult, confusing, and complicated disease.

THE DIAGNOSIS OF GBM OR HGG BEGINS A DIFFICULT JOURNEY FOR PATIENTS AND THEIR FAMILIES—A COMPLICATED JOURNEY FULL OF NEW PLACES, NEW STRESSORS AND ANXIETIES, A NEW LANGUAGE TO LEARN, AND NEW LIFE-ALTERING DECISIONS TO MAKE.

The diagnosis of GBM or HGG begins a difficult journey for patients and their families—a complicated journey full of new places, new stressors and anxieties, a new language to learn, and new life-altering decisions to make. Some patients and their families take a very passive role in their care, demonstrating an astounding amount of trust in their care team by cooperating with all our recommendations without question. For other patients and their families, the diagnosis of brain cancer becomes their new full-time job. They are determined to learn everything they can, to master all aspects of it, and to comprehensively weigh all decisions and options regarding testing and treatment. They are determined to exert as much control as possible over a situation that they feel they have no control over.

Julie was determined to understand and control as much of Kevin's future as she could. Unfortunately, a book like this didn't exist for Julie at that time. She was left to do most of her own research, ask dozens of questions, and take pages of notes during the limited time she had with Kevin's doctors. She traveled from Kentucky to Arizona and Tennessee for second and third opinions, trying to understand this terrible disease and be armed with the best knowledge so that she and Kevin could make the best decisions. She joined support groups for brain cancer and reached out to other patients and their families.

The purpose of this book is to provide people who are facing GBM or HGG, much like Julie and her husband, with a starting point to understand what to expect on this journey and a reference point they can always return to when the road changes and new challenges arise.

Throughout this book I will try to paint a picture of the journey the patient and their family will be traveling. I will try to anticipate and answer the common questions and challenges that will arise. I will try to simplify, guide, and aid in navigation through the complexities and decision-making involved with the diagnosis of GBM or HGG.

This book is also written to arm the reader with a knowledge and understanding of GBM and HGG so that everyone involved can be an effective and positive member of the patient's care and support team. Because every patient is different and every tumor has its subtle differences, this book is not meant to replace the expert advice of your care team but rather add to your understanding of GBM and HGG.

CHAPTER 1

WHAT IS GLIOBLASTOMA MULTIFORME? IT IS A BEAST ...

What exactly is cancer, and what does it mean to the patient?

What is the difference between glioblastoma and high-grade glioma?

How is glioblastoma or high-grade glioma different from other cancers?

Why are glioblastoma and high-grade glioma so difficult to treat?

If you are reading this book, it is probably because you, or someone you love, has just received news that no one wants to hear.

A mass has been found in their brain, and it's cancer.

So, what is cancer? And what does it mean if you have brain cancer?

Cancer, in general, is simply defined as a condition where a normal cell in your body decides it is going to multiply uncontrollably in such a manner that it will sicken the organ that it started in and possibly spread these uncontrolled cells to other parts of your body, which eventually also become sickened. If important or vital organs become involved, survival is in jeopardy.

TYPES OF BRAIN TUMORS

In the brain you can have two broad categories of tumor. The first is *primary*, which means that the tumor or cancer started in the brain, stays in the brain, and almost never spreads anywhere else. The second is *secondary*, which means that you've got cancer somewhere else in your body (lung, breast, colon, for example) and it has now spread to your brain.

Glioblastoma multiforme and high-grade glioma are the most serious forms of *primary* brain cancer. You should become familiar with the abbreviation GBM, because no one calls it glioblastoma multiforme. It's way too difficult to say. High-grade glioma is often abbreviated HGG.

TYPES OF GLIOMAS

Naming and classifying tumors is complex and often confusing to a patient. When you are initially diagnosed with a brain tumor, a piece of the tumor will be sent to a doctor called a pathologist who will issue a report. Within the report describing your tumor, you may see different types of brain cells mentioned. Your brain has only a few types of cells: neurons, ependymal cells, cells associated with blood vessels, and glial cells. A tumor involving glial cells is a glioma.

Gliomas may consist of several cell types. GBM and HGG are types of glioma that originate from a glial cell called an astrocyte. GBM and HGG occur when an astrocyte multiplies uncontrollably. Unlike other cancers, GBM and HGG do not spread to other organs in the body but can spread within the brain and, more rarely, the spine.

The World Health Organization (WHO) publishes a grading criterion for all types of tumors and cancers, including tumors of the brain and nervous system. According to WHO guidelines, tumors that come from astrocytes are divided into grades *I, II, III, IV*, with *I* and *II* being the least aggressive, or "low grade," and *III* and *IV* being the most aggressive, or "high grade."

Glioblastoma is a grade *IV* astrocytoma and the most aggressive type. High-grade glioma is grade *III*.

THE DIFFERENCE BETWEEN GLIOBLASTOMA AND HIGH-GRADE GLIOMA

The information provided in this book applies to *both* patients diagnosed with a WHO grade IV glioblastoma and WHO grade III high-grade glioma. While GBM and HGG are classified differently by the WHO, they are treated identically according to current guidelines. The difference between GBM and HGG concerns certain very specific microscopic characteristics that determine how aggressive a cancer is. An HGG does not have all the characteristics of a GBM and therefore is considered a less aggressive form of brain cancer. However, the recommendations for treatments, such as surgery, chemotherapy, and radiation, are the same.

GENETIC MARKERS

Research is occurring at cancer research centers to examine and understand the role of genetic mutations and gene sequencing in GBM and HGG. Genetic mutations have been found in these types of tumors, and research is ongoing to identify treatment strategies. Your doctor may order a molecular test of your tumor tissue, called a *biomarker*, to see if your tumor contains any mutations or particular genetic characteristics. Although advances are being made in understanding the genetics, there is still much to learn regarding the value of the information. At this time, the usefulness of this information to determine better treatment strategies is still evolving.

THE CHALLENGE OF TREATING GBM AND HGG

When I began my career as a neurosurgeon, my partner and I were talking about the management of a new GBM patient. He said to me, "I started practicing neurosurgery in 1973, and we're almost no better at treating this disease today than my first day in 1973." In many ways this statement is true, especially when compared to the progress made in the treatment of some other types of cancer.

> WHILE GBM AND HGG ARE NOT CONSIDERED "CURABLE" BY CANCER EXPERTS AT THIS TIME, THIS DISEASE CAN BE TREATED AGGRESSIVELY BY A VARIETY OF METHODS.

While GBM and HGG are not considered "curable" by cancer experts at this time, this disease can be treated aggressively by a variety of methods, which this book will review and explain. Hundreds of millions of dollars are being invested in research being done by hundreds of scientists across the world who have dedicated their entire careers to advancing the treatment of

GBM and HGG to find a treatment that will one day result in consistent long-term survival, if not a cure. In the time I've been a neurosurgeon, technological advances have been made in the diagnosis and treatment of GBM and HGG. Progress continues to be made on all fronts against this disease. And, of course, today we do see "long-term survivors" of GBM and HGG. Increasing numbers of patients have had amazing responses to treatment and have far outlived the normal course of the disease.

There's an old saying in golf that if you play golf long enough and often enough, statistics demonstrate that you will likely get a "hole in one" eventually. The same is said about neurosurgeons and GBM patients. Most neurosurgeons who have been practicing tumor surgery for a long time will eventually get their hole in one—a long-term GBM/HGG survivor that defies all the odds.

So, now is the part where you ask *why* the treatment of GBM and HGG is so challenging for physicians and clinical researchers. There are a couple of important things to understand about GBM/HGG and the brain that might shed some light on why this disease is so difficult to treat.

"Why can't you just cut it out?" Let me try to explain why it's so hard to remove a GBM/HGG as opposed to other brain tumors. Imagine that you have two bowls of cold Jell-O. The first bowl has a whole strawberry inside the Jell-O, about a quarter of an inch below the surface. Now I'm going to give you a butter knife and a small spoon and challenge you to take out the entire strawberry without disrupting or ruining any of the Jell-O around it. What do you think? Not impossible, and if I gave you a couple of bowls to practice on, I'd bet most people could do a good job of getting that strawberry out. That's what it's like to operate on every brain tumor ... *except* GBM/HGG.

Now imagine that a second bowl of Jell-O is made by putting a teaspoonful of whipped cream in while it was still liquid and swirled it around a little before putting the bowl in the refrigerator. Now I'm going to give you the same butter knife and small spoon and challenge you to take out all the whipped cream and disrupt or destroy as little of the Jell-O as possible. Now what do you think? Much harder, right? In fact, it is probably impossible to do it in most cases without significant damage to the surrounding Jell-O—and you still wouldn't get all the whipped cream out. That's what it's like to operate on GBM/HGG.

GBM and HGG penetrate into the brain tissue in such a way that removing all the cancerous cells during surgery is impossible for two reasons: number one, you can't see each and every tumor cell, and number two, even if you could, you'd likely cause a lot of damage to the brain trying to remove all the cancerous cells. The best we can hope for is to remove all the tumor seen on the MRI or other tumor-visualization technologies. But neurosurgeons know that we *always* leave cancerous cells behind.

You may wonder why chemotherapy or other medications don't kill those cancer cells left behind after surgery. The answer is an interesting piece of anatomy called the *blood-brain barrier*. Chemotherapy and medication travel to the site of a tumor/cancer through the bloodstream. For most cancers, blood vessels that feed the tumor also provide the route to deliver powerful chemotherapy and medication to destroy the tumor cells. Your brain, however, protects itself by creating a barrier that makes it difficult for medication to reach the brain tumor. This will be discussed more in chapter 6 when I describe how chemotherapy works.

The goal of this chapter is to provide a better understanding of what GBM and HGG are and why they can be difficult to treat. But the good news is that patients are not alone in this fight. Besides friends and family to offer their support and love, there is an entire team of new friends who have dedicated their lives to treating GBM/HGG, and we all will work tirelessly to help patients navigate this journey.

TAKEAWAYS:

- Cancer occurs when a cell in the body reproduces in an uncontrolled manner and causes organs and systems in the body to become diseased.

- Glioblastoma and high-grade glioma are both a primary cancer of the glial cells of the brain. HGG is a less aggressive form of brain cancer, but GBM and HGG are essentially treated the same.

- GBM and HGG are different from other cancers of the body in that they do not spread to other parts of the body.

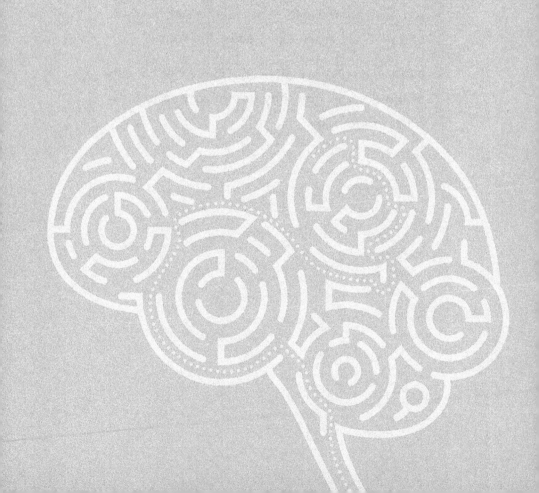

CHAPTER 2

YOUR TEAM

· ·

Who are the key players in my care?

What role will each key person play in my care?

In the emergency room, I was the first doctor to meet with Kevin and Julie and tell them about the results of the CT scans and MRI. From there, Kevin was admitted to the hospital and prepared for surgery the next day to remove his brain tumor. While in the hospital, Kevin and Julie had a steady stream of friends and family visiting. In fact, Kevin's friends and family created a schedule so that someone close to Kevin was always at his side both day and night.

Kevin was discharged home a few days later, but at that time we still didn't know that he had a GBM. It took the pathologists at our hospital and a specially trained neuropathologist at the Mayo Clinic in Minnesota about a week to report the final diagnosis of GBM.

Once the pathology report was received, we brought Kevin and Julie back to the cancer center to talk about his diagnosis of GBM. Kevin and Julie each brought their parents for support during this visit. At the end of this visit, they left with appointments to see our medical oncologist and radiation oncologist to start the next steps in Kevin's treatment.

Kevin's team started to get built immediately with his wife, Julie, in the emergency room. The next member added was me. His team grew during his stay in the hospital to include his friends and family who joined to help in his care and provide social and emotional support. Once he was back at home, the team continued to grow to include members he would never even meet personally, such as the pathologist working to help determine his diagnosis. By the time Kevin and Julie left my office a week or so after surgery, the team that had been built to guide, support, and shepherd them through the diagnosis of GBM had grown into dozens of people.

For GBM/HGG treatment, you or your loved one will have an oncology team that will be there to support you at *every step* of this journey. Of course, this team will consist of several medical and healthcare specialists, but it also may include nonmedical members who will be equally as important. Depending on your needs at any given time, the number that you interact with regularly will change. As few as three or more than twenty might be members of your team.

This is primarily because decisions regarding your care are a team effort and not directed by only one person. Some cancer centers have a dedicated tumor board or will conduct a treatment-planning conference that consists of the key cancer experts. Each member of this group brings their unique knowledge, experience, and perspective. These experts discuss each patient, the details of the patient's tumor, and the patient's health situation. They consider all available treatment options and make recommendations for treatment. These groups meet regularly to discuss patients. These members will also consult each other *informally* when new patient issues arise.

THE NEUROSURGEON

You have already met the leader of the team, the neurosurgeon. While each member of the team will play an important role in your care and treatment, your neurosurgeon will take the lead to coordinate your care.

When you experienced the first signs or symptoms that something was wrong with your health, you may have gone to see your primary care doctor, or perhaps you went to an emergency room. One of those doctors ordered a CT or MRI test of your head. The test revealed an abnormal growth on your brain. When the doctor saw the result of that test, their next action was to send you to see a neurosurgeon. Your neurosurgeon explained that the only way to know what that abnormal growth was, and to make a diagnosis, was to take a piece of it out during an operation.

All neurosurgeons are trained to take out brain tumors, but not all neurosurgeons will specialize in brain tumor treatment. Like many other jobs, medical professionals tend to narrow down the scope of their job to become experts in one area or another. For example, some lawyers focus on criminal law while some prefer family law. Some car mechanics specialize in foreign cars, some on large trucks. Neurosurgeons are no different. Some neurosurgeons focus on diseases of the spine and arthritis conditions, some focus on the blood vessels that feed the brain and spine, and some focus on cancer and tumors.

Your neurosurgeon should be someone who makes removing and treating brain tumors a significant part of their practice—meaning someone who treats a large number of brain tumor patients and takes a special interest in cancer and the complexities presented by cancer and cancer treatment. The brain tumor neurosurgeon is also likely to work at a hospital that has access to the needed specialists and the most up-to-date equipment for the treatment of brain tumors. Your neurosurgeon will perform the surgery to remove the tumor, and they will follow you through the whole course of your treatment and recovery. Typically, you will meet with your neurosurgeon about every three months to review the results of the latest testing and discuss how you're doing. Your neurosurgeon will *always* be a part of your treatment team.

THE MEDICAL ONCOLOGIST OR NEURO-ONCOLOGIST

These specialists are internal medicine doctors who have had several extra years of specialty education in cancer care. Many medical oncologists treat a variety of different cancers, but in some places you will see a *neuro*-oncologist. This is an oncologist who has narrowed their practice to the medical treatment of brain tumors.

Medical oncologists, or neuro-oncologists, are experts in the non-surgical treatment of cancer. Their role in your care is to determine whether chemotherapy, immunotherapy, and other medication-type treatments will effectively treat the cancer. These therapies are intended to kill cancer cells and stop them from multiplying and spreading to other parts of the body. The oncologist prescribes the chemotherapy medication and will manage any side effects that you may have. Medical oncologists are associated with a cancer center or a hospital that has an *infusion center*. An infusion center is a facility designed to prepare the medications and is staffed by certified registered nurses who will give the chemotherapy or immunotherapy to the patients. Depending on the type of chemotherapy that you receive, you may see the oncologist once per week or once per month. A GBM/HGG patient will typically meet with their oncologist about once a month.

THE RADIATION ONCOLOGIST

The radiation oncologist is a doctor who has had special training in the use of radiation to treat many different types of cancer and tumors. Radiation treatment for a GBM is part of the standard initial treatment.

The radiation oncologist works in a *radiation center* that is often part of a larger cancer center or hospital. The radiation oncologist is an expert in the delivery of radiation treatments for cancer. They create a personal radiation treatment plan for each patient that takes into account the type of tumor, the size of the tumor, and the location of the tumor. Because there are several types of radiation treatments and radiation machines, the radiation oncologist determines which method of delivery will be most effective to treat your cancer and minimize possible side effects.

Once the radiation treatments are complete, you may not see the radiation oncologist often, but they remain part of your treatment team and continue to provide input and offer treatment recommendations.

THE RADIOLOGIST

A radiologist is a doctor who is trained to read, interpret, and report on all of the different imaging and X-ray studies that are being done. This includes MRIs, CT scans, plain X-rays, nuclear medicine images, plus many more. The radiologist may perform procedures that use imaging to improve the accuracy of a procedure. They may also insert special intravenous lines that will be used to give the chemotherapy and other medication. While all radiologists are trained to read MRIs and interpret brain imaging, some radiologists receive specialized training in the brain and spine. These doctors are called *neuroradiologists*. Most cancer centers that treat a large number of brain tumor patients have the expertise of a neuroradiologist available. In GBM and HGG, the radiologist reads and interprets MRI scans of the brain to assess progress and the effect of treatments and to watch for the tumor returning.

As a patient, you may not meet with the radiologist, but they are members of the treatment team and participate in the meetings to give their expert opinion on the MRI and suggest other imaging methods that may be helpful.

THE PATHOLOGIST

The pathologist is a doctor who specializes in the microscopic, molecular, and genetic analysis of tissue and blood samples from the body. What does that mean to the patient? The tumor from your brain or the biopsy sample is sent to the pathologist, who looks at it under a microscope and performs tests to determine if your tumor is a GBM, an HGG, a lower-grade glioma, or a tumor from a cancer elsewhere in the body (metastasis), such as lung cancer.

Just like all the other doctors described in this chapter, pathologists can also specialize. Those who have had specialized training in diseases of the brain and spine are called *neuropathologists*. Neuro-pathologists are not common, and there are only a handful in the country. Most are at major university centers that do scientific brain cancer research. Therefore, it is common for community hospitals and cancer centers to send the tumor tissue samples to a university center to be evaluated by a neuropathologist for a second opinion or a more in-depth evaluation.

As a patient, you will never meet your pathologist, but they, too, are part of your treatment team and will meet with the other professionals to help evaluate your tumor. Your oncologist may make decisions about the type of chemotherapy you receive based on the pathologist's report of your tumor and its particular characteristics.

THE REGISTERED NURSE

The neurosurgeon, medical oncologist, and radiation oncologists all have oncology registered nurses who work in their practices. Oncology nurses are often certified as oncology RNs and have several years of experience caring for cancer patients. You may see the nurse before you meet with the doctor when you go to your appointments. The nurse will inquire as to how you are feeling, what symptoms you are having, and what medications you are taking, and they may also check your weight, temperature, blood pressure, and heart rate. They will communicate this information to the doctor. RNs are sometimes called nurse navigators, and they are the liaison with the doctor and will help you manage symptoms, coordinate appointments, and communicate your information to the doctors quickly and thoroughly. They will educate you as to how to prepare for and what to expect from surgery, radiation, and chemotherapy treatments.

OTHER MEMBERS OF THE TEAM

In addition to providing all the necessary medical and nursing experts to treat cancer, cancer centers also provide a wide variety of other experts to support you and help you throughout your treatment. Examples include clinical dieticians, genetic counselors, patient advocates and navigators, financial counselors, and social workers.

The diagnosis of any cancer is a life-changing event for all patients. Cancer affects not only the patient but also their family, finances, job, relationships, and even their faith.

Most cancer centers recognize the far-reaching effects of a cancer diagnosis and offer services to support the patient during this trying and difficult time.

Nutritionist/dietician. Oncology professionals are recognizing more and more the benefit of nutritional support as an adjunct therapy for the cancer patient. Data supports the importance of good nutrition before, during, and following cancer treatments. It is in your best interest as a cancer patient when undergoing treatment to stay healthy and well nourished to optimize your quality of life during treatment and after. A more specific discussion of the role of diet in GBM and HGG will be discussed in later chapters.

Genetic counselor. Cancer is like looking at a menu at an ice cream shop. Everything on the menu is ice cream, but there are dozens of flavors and types. Cancer isn't one disease—it's hundreds of different diseases. The more we learn of the defects and mutations in the genetic code of cancer DNA, the more the number of flavors on the menu just increases. As genetic science has progressed, GBM and HGG have been subclassified depending on what type of genetic profile your particular tumor has (what particular nuts, fruits, and flavors are in your ice cream). This genetic profile is increasingly becoming a factor in how your GBM/HGG is treated. Genetic counselors can help the patient and family understand these genetic factors and how they determine treatment. In other types of cancer, such as certain types of breast cancer, genetic counselors play an important role in advising families of how cancer risk factors can be passed on to other family members. This is *not true* of GBM and HGG. Currently there is no inherited risk factor for GBM and HGG that we know about.

Patient advocate/navigator. The patient advocate or patient navigator is a nonmedical member or a volunteer whose job is to help the patient manage the hospital and medical system. They can help you contact offices, make appointments, organize your treatments, arrange transportation or lodging, or help with parking. Very often the navigators are persons who themselves are cancer survivors and have been patients at the cancer center where you are being treated. They are familiar with the center, the staff, the challenges of arranging appointments, and, importantly, the wide range of emotions that patients experience.

Chaplain/priest/minister. Spirituality and religious beliefs are very important to some people but not as important to others. Most cancer centers recognize the role of spirituality for the patient, and chaplain services and spiritual guidance are often available during their care. It is also not unusual for patients and families to bring their own spiritual or religious advisor to their medical appointments for emotional support and guidance.

Financial counselor. The complexities of insurance, benefits, billing, and copays can become overwhelming to patients and their families. Cancer centers will have financial counselors available to patients to help them navigate these issues. More information about this will be covered in a later chapter.

Family and friends. The value of the involvement of family and friends cannot be overstated on this journey. At any given medical appointment, the amount of information that is discussed and the decisions that need to be considered can be overwhelming to the patient. The presence of a friend or family member who can keep notes, provide emotional support, and act as another set of eyes and ears can be very helpful. Patients may be recovering from physical disabilities and require help with normal activities such as cooking, dressing, shopping, or driving. I can't recall ever seeing a GBM patient "go it alone." This is not a condition you can keep to yourself. At times, the patient will need time alone to process and cope with their condition, and at times well-intentioned friends and family may overwhelm a situation, but the opportunity to share your care and the steps along this journey with the people in your life who love you is essential to your recovery as well as to their own psychological well-being.

TAKEAWAYS:

- The treatment and management of GBM as a team will include many dedicated people, from doctors and nutritionists to loved ones and friends.

- Each member of your team and family will play an important role in managing your care or supporting you through this journey.

CHAPTER 3

IMAGING TESTS

What's the difference between a CT scan and an MRI?

Why do I have to get imaging so frequently?

How do you know if the tumor is coming back or growing?

I met with Kevin and Julie about every ten to twelve weeks in my office. Almost every visit started with Kevin and Julie registering at our imaging center to get an MRI of the brain. Once the MRI was completed, they would come over to my office for their appointment to discuss how Kevin was doing and review the results of the MRI.

These are generally stressful visits for the patient and their family because the MRI is the best tool to measure the effectiveness of the surgery, chemotherapy, and radiation. The result of the MRI may tell us if the cancer is under control or not.

The minute I walked into that exam room, Julie wanted my assessment of the MRI. She didn't want to say, "Hello—how are you?

Nice weather we're having. How was your weekend?"—nothing. Just "Sit down and tell us what the MRI shows."

CT SCAN

Anyone with a GBM diagnosis will have many scans, also called diagnostic images, of their brain. There are a few ways to image the brain, the two most common being a CT scan, which is shorthand for computerized tomography, and an MRI, which stands for magnetic resonance imaging. The first test a patient will experience is typically a plain CT scan of the brain. This is usually done when someone complains of worsening headaches, weakness in an arm or leg, a new episode of confusion, or a seizure. A CT scan is a large, powerful X-ray computer that circles around the patient and creates three-dimensional (3D) pictures or images. CT is wonderful for imaging bone and can be very helpful imaging organs in the chest and abdomen. CT scans are good tests to detect things such as swelling or bleeding in the brain, and they can be very useful to find injuries when a person has been in an accident such as a car crash or a fall. A plain CT of the brain, however, does not provide a lot of detail. It's kind of like watching an old black-and-white television with bad reception. You can tell something is there, but you may not be sure what you're seeing. CT machines are fast and cost effective, and every emergency room has one available day and night, so it is often the first test you'll have.

When a GBM or HGG is present, though, a plain CT will most often show a fuzzy mass and swelling, which is just enough information to tell your doctor that there is something abnormal and that you need an MRI of your brain.

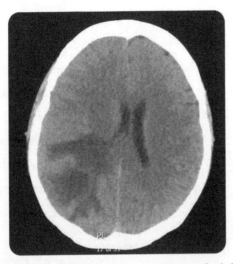

*CT scan of the brain showing a tumor on the left side
of the page and dark area of brain swelling around it.*

MRI SCAN

An MRI is a much more useful and detailed test. If the CT scan is like
an old black-and-white TV, then an MRI is like a 4K high-definition
flat screen! The doctor will probably order an MRI of the brain with
contrast, because it is the best way to see any brain tumor.

An MRI provides a high-quality, detailed image of your brain
and the tumor, but it does *not* tell us exactly what we're seeing on the
scan. Many different diseases of the brain can imitate a tumor on an
MRI, such as an infection or diseases such as multiple sclerosis. Only
the biopsy can properly identify a GBM/HGG tumor.

The MRI of the brain takes more time to do than a CT scan,
and the MRI machine makes more noise than the CT scanner. Some
people do not like to be in small spaces and may feel claustrophobic
when inside the MRI scanner. Medication can be used to help them
relax during this time.

Once a GBM diagnosis has been made, MRI scans of the brain will be needed every eight to sixteen weeks. The frequency will be determined by your team based on the results of the previous scan and whether any new neurologic symptoms occur. The purpose of the frequent MRIs is to check the effect of treatment and to monitor for new tumor growth or recurrence. The team will monitor brain tumors very closely with frequent scans so that any new growth is caught very early, when it is small.

THE PURPOSE OF THE FREQUENT MRIs IS TO CHECK THE EFFECT OF TREATMENT AND TO MONITOR FOR NEW TUMOR GROWTH OR RECURRENCE.

The doctor will order an "MRI with contrast." What is contrast? Contrast is a substance called *gadolinium*. It is injected through a vein in your arm. The MRI scan will create a series of pictures of the brain before the contrast is injected, followed by a series of pictures after the contrast is injected. The contrast will cause the solid parts of a GBM and the outer edges to "light up" or "*enhance*," differentiating it from normal brain tissue. You will hear your team mention and talk about this *enhancement* on the MRI. It is this enhancement on the MRI that may signal new tumor growth or recurrence.

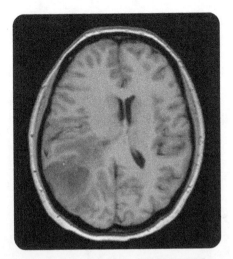

MRI scan of the brain done WITHOUT contrast showing a tumor on the left side of the page.

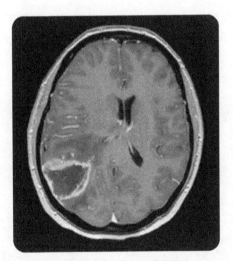

Same MRI scan of the brain WITH contrast. You can now see the "Ring" of enhancement that identifies the tumor.

While enhancement can be worrisome, not all enhancement indicates that there is a tumor. Scar tissue after surgery and the effect of radiation treatments can also cause brain tissue to enhance. This is called *pseudoprogression* or *false progression*. False progression can look exactly like tumor growth but could be due to the effects of radiation or surgery.

DIFFERENT TYPES OF MRI SCANS

A couple of special MRI scans may be used to try to determine true tumor growth versus false progression. The first is a *magnetic resonance spectroscopy*, or MRS. MRS can be used to help determine if changes on the MRI are due to growth of the tumor or the result of radiation or an infection. The MRS measures certain "chemical signatures" in your brain. These chemical signatures can then be compared to the known signatures seen in GBM, radiated tissue, and infection. Think of it as a magnetic biopsy that can help your treatment team make decisions.

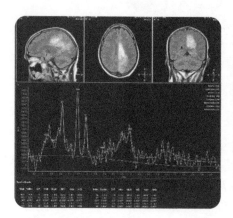 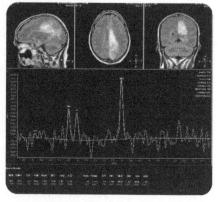

MR spectroscopy of the brain. The image on the left of the page shows a high spike on the graph indicating tumor. The image on the right of the page shows a high spike on the graph indicating normal brain.

Another special MRI scan that may be used is a *magnetic resonance perfusion*, or MRP. MRP measures how fast and how much blood is flowing to a particular part of your brain. A growing tumor will have more blood flow compared to normal brain tissue while false progression from radiation will typically show less blood flow compared to normal brain tissue.

Sometimes even these special MRI scans are not enough to determine what the changes on the MRI mean and a biopsy or more surgery is needed to get tissue samples.

An additional type of MRI that may be used is a *functional MRI*, or fMRI. This type of MRI scan is not used to decide whether your tumor has changed in size. It is used to help your surgeon plan for surgery. Functional MRI provides a map of the critical areas of your brain and color codes those areas so that your surgeon has a picture of where the tumor is in relation to those critical areas such as speech, language, or the part of your brain that controls your arms and legs. This may help your surgeon avoid these important areas when removing the tumor. During an fMRI, the patient lies in the MRI machine and is asked to do a series of specific tests or actions while the machine is scanning your brain. You may be asked to tap your toes or wiggle your hands and fingers. You also may be asked to look at a screen and play word games silently in your head while the machine is scanning. By doing these movements and activities during the scan, the computer will build a color-coded map that shows the surgeon which part of the brain controls those actions. Not every patient will need an fMRI. If the neurosurgeon already knows that the tumor is not in a critical area of the brain, surgery can proceed safely without the information an fMRI provides.

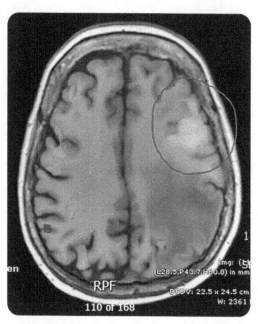

Functional MRI image of the brain. The area circled shows the critical language area activated during a word task.

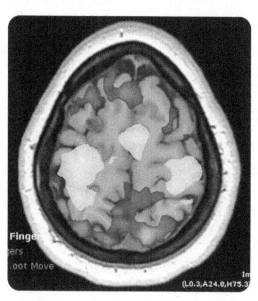

Functional MRI image of the brain. The lighter areas to the left and right show activation of the parts of the brain responsible for finger movement.

TAKEAWAYS:

- A CT scan is a quick look at your brain that provides limited information about the brain. An MRI is a longer imaging study that provides a very detailed image of the brain.

- GBM patients will be imaged about every twelve weeks to assess how effective treatment is and to look for early changes.

- Changes on an MRI will usually be the first way you will discover that the tumor is coming back.

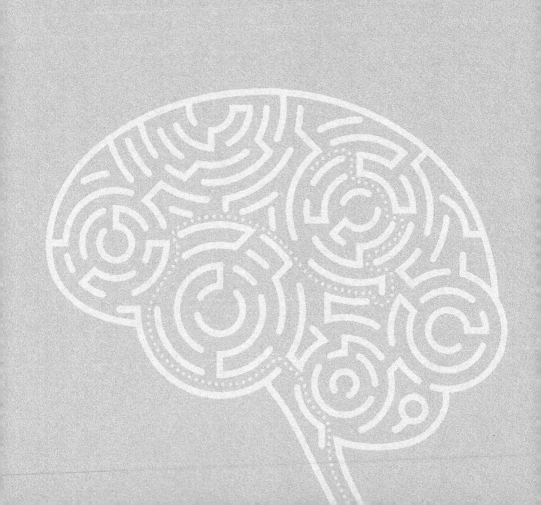

CHAPTER 4

THE COOKBOOK

· ·

> What or who determines what treatment is done for GBM?
>
> What happens if a treatment appears not to be working?

We are always very supportive of our patients seeking a second opinion when they get a life-altering diagnosis such as GBM and HGG. For example, Kevin was a young man in the prime of his life when he received his diagnosis. It was going to be very important for him and his family to feel confident that they were getting the best available care moving forward.

We arranged to have Kevin and Julie seen at two other major university centers considered leaders in the treatment of GBM. They returned from these appointments slightly surprised but satisfied when they learned that the treatment they had already received at our cancer center and the treatment we had planned going forward was exactly what the major university centers recommended. That's when I explained to them that every cancer center worked from the same "cookbook" or "playbook," known as the NCCN Guidelines.

THE NATIONAL COMPREHENSIVE CANCER NETWORK

The National Comprehensive Cancer Network (NCCN) is an alliance of the most notable Comprehensive Cancer Centers in the country. One of the NCCN's core purposes is the publication and frequent updating of the NCCN Clinical Practice Guidelines. These guidelines are the "cookbook" for cancer care and are written by experts from around the world who use the latest medical and scientific knowledge and expert opinion to provide diagnostic and treatment recommendations for many types of cancer. The *NCCN Guidelines for Physicians* is an excellent publication, and any member of your team of specialists may mention it to you. The cancer committee or tumor board will likely use the NCCN Guidelines for GBM and HGG as their signpost for the majority of your treatment decisions. The guidelines spell out the courses of treatment recommended for GBM and HGG.

NCCN also provides information for patients and families to help them learn about their diagnoses and treatments. The patient information is on the NCCN website (www.nccn.org). For GBM and HGG information, you can go to the website, click the link for *NCCN Guidelines for Patients*, and enter the words *brain cancer* in the search field. You will be able to download the guidelines as a PDF, or you can read the document on your computer. The NCCN mentions several treatments and provides facts about several types of brain tumors, but many patients find the information to be too general and not helpful enough to answer their many questions. This is one of the reasons this book was written—to provide more useful information to patients and their families as they go through this journey.

No publication or set of guidelines will cover every possible situation that a patient may face. A person's tumor might progress to a point where the NCCN Guidelines reach the end of the approved recommendations. This does not necessarily mean the patient is completely out of all treatment options. Very often a patient may move through all the standard treatments of surgery, radiation, and multiple types of chemotherapy outlined in the NCCN Guidelines, and recurrence or progression of the tumor occurs. If the patient is feeling well and functioning well, then this is when you will rely on the experience and expertise of your team of specialists and the cancer committee to decide what the next step in treatment is, understanding that treatments at this point may not be standard and often may involve clinical experimental trials. This is also the point at which a second opinion may be helpful to explore other nonstandard or experimental clinical trials available at other centers.

Because the NCCN relies on scientific evidence and expert opinion, you will *not* find any information in the NCCN Guidelines about experimental, holistic, or any other treatments that have not been rigorously evaluated according to scientific principles.

THE KARNOFSKY PERFORMANCE SCALE

The *NCCN Guidelines for Physicians* uses something called the Karnofsky Performance Scale. This scale assesses the patient's overall ability to function in everyday activities and is used to determine a patient's ability to tolerate treatment. The Karnofsky Performance Scale runs from zero to one hundred, with one hundred being "normal." The *NCCN Guidelines for Physicians* uses a cutoff of sixty to guide physician decision-making during treatments. If a GBM patient can bathe themselves, cook for themselves, be left alone, and walk without falling down, they are above a sixty. The Karnofsky scale is an efficient way to communicate how functional the patient is with one number.

KARNOFSKY PERFORMANCE SCALE

DEFINITION		INDEX DESCRIPTION
Able to carry on normal activity and to work. No special care is needed.	100	Normal; no complaints; no evidence of disease.
	90	Able to carry on normal activity; minor signs or symptoms of disease.
	80	Normal activity with effort; some signs or symptoms of disease.
Unable to work. Able to live at home, care for most personal needs. A varying amount of assistance is needed.	70	Cares for self. Unable to carry on normal activity or do active work.
	60	Requires occasional assistance, but is able to care for most of his needs.
	50	Requires considerable assistance and frequent medical care.
Unable to care for self. Requires equivalent of institutional or hospital care. Disease may be progressing rapidly.	40	Disabled; requires special care and assistance.
	30	Severely disabled; hospitalization indicated although death not imminent.
	20	Very sick; hospitalization necessary; active supportive treatment necessary.
	10	Moribund; fatal processes progressing rapidly.
	0	Dead

The important point I am making here is that a patient's eligibility for treatment will depend on what the MRI shows and how the tumor is behaving, but it also may depend upon the overall health and condition of the patient. A fifty-year-old healthy marathon runner with a GBM is in a much better position to recover from surgery and tolerate chemotherapy and radiation and manage any side effects or disabilities compared to a fifty-year-old patient with emphysema and diabetes who is eighty pounds overweight and is already using a walker.

A PATIENT'S ELIGIBILITY FOR TREATMENT WILL DEPEND ON WHAT THE MRI SHOWS AND HOW THE TUMOR IS BEHAVING, BUT IT ALSO MAY DEPEND UPON THE OVERALL HEALTH AND CONDITION OF THE PATIENT.

TAKEAWAYS:

- NCCN Guidelines provide the medical community a single source for the standard accepted care and treatment for GBM and HGG.

- If it appears that treatment is not working, then your treatment team will meet to discuss the next treatments based on their experience, NCCN Guidelines, and best medical evidence.

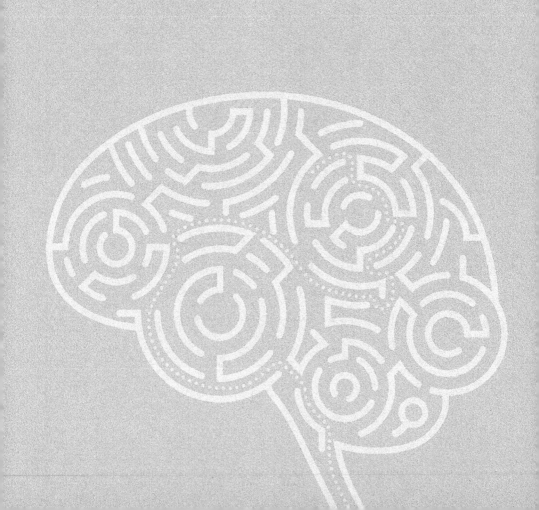

CHAPTER 5

SURGERY

· ·

> Why is surgery for GBM so important?
>
> Do I need a biopsy, or can we just take the whole tumor out?
>
> What can I expect through my experience with surgery?

From the emergency room, Kevin was admitted into the hospital. He underwent some initial testing that is done for all patients with a new tumor, was started on steroids for his brain swelling, and was given an antiseizure medicine. He was scheduled for a surgery called a craniotomy the next day.

The following day, Kevin underwent surgery to the right frontal part of his brain. Thankfully the tumor was in a part of Kevin's brain that did not control any vital functions, and I was able to remove all of the tumor seen on the MRI.

Kevin was moved to the intensive care unit to be watched closely by the nursing staff and to recover overnight. The next day Kevin felt strong and was having no complications from the surgery. He underwent a postsurgery MRI and was carefully assisted by our physical therapists to get up and out of his hospital bed. Two days later he was discharged to return home with Julie.

THE FIRST STEP: SURGERY

Every GBM/HGG story starts with surgery. In fact, if you're reading this book, you may already have had surgery. The tumor tissue obtained during that surgery is how the GBM or HGG diagnosis was made.

At this time, you may be asking, "What type of surgery did I have, and why?" In general, there are two ways to get a tissue sample from a brain tumor. The first option is a *biopsy*. A brain biopsy is done "stereotactically," meaning a guidance system is used to accurately direct the surgeon to the tumor. The brain biopsy is done through a small hole made in the skull, through which a thin biopsy probe about the size of a piece of spaghetti is passed into the tumor with the help and guidance of a computer system. The probe then takes out six to twelve rice-sized pieces of the tumor.

Similar to using the GPS in your car, your surgeon tells the computer where the biopsy probe is starting and then tells it where he or she wants the biopsy probe to go. This method is safe, accurate, and effective.

Because a biopsy removes only very small pieces of a tumor, the majority of the tumor, about 99 percent of it, is still in your head. The second option is a *craniotomy*. A craniotomy is a bigger operation where your surgeon makes a larger hole in your skull, maybe the size of a cookie. The goal of a craniotomy is to safely remove as much of the tumor as possible, also called a *gross total resection*.

BIOPSY OR CRANIOTOMY?

There are two reasons to do the craniotomy and remove as much tumor tissue as possible rather than just a biopsy. The first is to relieve the patient's neurologic symptoms that are caused by the tumor. Removing as much of the tumor tissue as possible will reduce brain swelling and take pressure off the normal structures of the brain, which often can improve the neurologic problems being caused by the tumor. The second reason to do a craniotomy rather than a biopsy is that for most brain tumors, removing as much tumor tissue as possible with surgery is also the best way to control and treat the tumor.

So why would my surgeon *just* do a biopsy and not take the whole tumor out right away? Good question. There are a few reasons. If your tumor is in a critical location of your brain that controls speech and language function, then a biopsy to establish a diagnosis might be a reasonable first step rather than jumping into a larger craniotomy and risking damage to an area of critical function. Another reason is that some tumors are located in parts of the brain where removing them could result in permanent coma or even death. Certain diagnoses may not require a large craniotomy and a biopsy is used just to establish an exact diagnosis so that more informed treatment decisions can be made. The most common reason a biopsy is done is that the tumor cannot be safely removed, either because of its size or its location.

Here are two patient examples to illustrate when a craniotomy is appropriate and when a biopsy is preferred. I have a patient who was diagnosed with GBM in the front of the brain, on the right side, just above the right eye. Fortunately, this part of the brain is not responsible for critical or lifesaving functions. I like to call it "optional equipment." Life is better if you have them, but a person can have a pretty normal life without them. This patient's GBM has recurred twice, and he had three uncomplicated craniotomies and recovered well. Each time, the MRI shows no remaining tumor. Because the tumor keeps recurring in the right frontal lobe (an area of the brain with no critical functions), we can do extensive surgery in this area and not worry about causing any neurologic problems.

I have another patient who presented with a tumor deep in the left part of his brain called the *thalamus*. The thalamus is a small structure about four inches deep in our brain. We need the thalamus to function normally. It's what a real estate agent might call a "high-priced location." The part of the brain in and around the thalamus acts as an important relay center for the nerve connections between your brain and the rest of your body. A stereotactic biopsy was decided upon, as it was the safest way to determine the diagnosis without causing a serious neurologic problem.

In many cases of a new tumor, a patient will undergo a full craniotomy rather than a biopsy because no matter what kind of tumor it is, it's best to remove as much of the tumor as safely as possible. In the process, the pressure on the brain that is caused by the tumor is relieved, and most often the patients will feel better and function better after surgery. The diagnosis can then be made from the tumor tissue that was removed.

WHY SURGERY IS SO IMPORTANT

In GBM and HGG, surgery is considered the *most important* factor to control the tumor and will have the biggest impact on the patient's survival. Current medical literature points toward removing as much of the tumor as seen on the MRI as safely as possible. Exactly how much tumor should be removed is a matter of debate by experts around the world. Some studies have shown a maximum survival benefit when 98 percent of the tumor is removed. Most new and emerging surgical technology and research are geared toward developing tools and techniques to remove all of the tumor tissue that is seen on the various medical images. What we do know is that if your postoperative MRI doesn't show any tumor tissue or very little tumor tissue, you're going to do better than if, for example, 50 percent of the tumor is left behind.

IN GBM AND HGG, SURGERY IS CONSIDERED THE MOST IMPORTANT FACTOR TO CONTROL THE TUMOR AND WILL HAVE THE BIGGEST IMPACT ON THE PATIENT'S SURVIVAL.

SURGICAL TOOLS

Different cancer centers will invest in different technologies to aid in the safe and maximum amount of tumor removal. The ongoing question is this: Which of these technologies is "best"? Since *best* is difficult to quantify, I'm going to refrain from recommending any one technology. Instead, I'm going to describe the different tools your surgeon may use so you can better understand what may be available. Your neurosurgeon should discuss the options with you as well as the pros and cons of each technique or technology.

STEREOTACTIC NAVIGATION

We've already touched on this during the biopsy section of this book. Stereotactic guidance for brain surgery is the absolute minimal standard of care for any tumor removal. Your surgeon should *at least* be using a computer-guided stereotactic navigation system to aid in removing your tumor and also when performing a biopsy.

Think of stereotactic navigation as a GPS for brain surgery. It's a computer display in the operating room that shows the surgeon the MRI of the brain and tells the surgeon precisely where they are in the brain during surgery. This allows the surgeon to make as small an incision as possible, at the exact location of the tumor. It also allows the surgeon to select a route to the tumor that is the shortest distance, or a route that will avoid critical brain tissue and disturb as little of the normal brain as possible. Stereotactic navigation makes removing the maximum amount of the tumor more likely with fewer complications.

FUNCTIONAL MRI

A *functional MRI*, or fMRI, is an imaging scan done before surgery. It creates a color-coded map that shows the location of the tumor and the critical areas of brain function for the surgeon (see chapter 3, "Imaging Tests," for a more in-depth description).

INTRAOPERATIVE MRI

An *intraoperative MRI* is a special operating room that has been built with an MRI scanner in the room that can be used during surgery. This allows the surgeon to do an MRI scan during the operation so they can be confident they have removed all of the tumor that can be seen on the MRI.

Hospitals with intraoperative MRI scanners are not widely available because of the extraordinary cost of building such a facility. In addition, while brain tumor centers that regularly use intraoperative MRI report that they can remove *more* of the tumor, how *much* more, and whether this translates into achieving a longer life for the patient, is controversial.

FLUORESCENCE

Another innovation in GBM surgery is the ability to cause the tumor to "light up" during surgery so that hidden parts of the tumor can be seen with special lights and filters through a surgical microscope. Technology that allows a tumor to light up has been used to treat other cancers besides GBM/HGG for years. However, only recently has a technique been developed to apply this technology to GBM surgery.

Gleolan, or 5-aminolevulinic acid (5-ALA), is a solution the patient drinks three to six hours before brain surgery. Once the surgeon has the tumor and brain in view, they can look through the surgical microscope or specialized eyewear with a special light and light filter, and the GBM/HGG tissue will glow a pinkish orange while the normal brain glows a bluish color. The 5-ALA solution is absorbed only by GBM/HGG tissue and not normal brain tissue. This allows the surgeon to see *more* of the areas that are involved with a tumor than they would ordinarily see.

While we know 5-ALA is safe and will often result in a larger amount of GBM/HGG tissue being removed during surgery, how much and whether this translates into the patient living longer is an area of ongoing research.

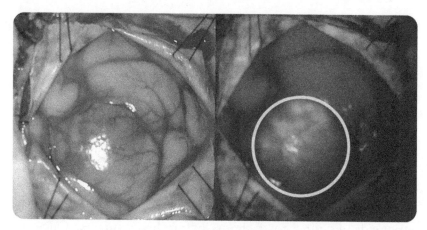

Image from surgery on the left is without 5-ALA and viewing filter. Image on the right is after 5-ALA is given viewed through the filter. The 5ALA causes the area within the white circle to appear pink to the surgeon. Image obtained from the applicant-submitted protocol for fluorescence-guided resection of high-grade (grade IV) glioma that are glioblastoma multiforme (GBM) using oral aminolevulonic acid hydrochloride (ALA), Medical Services Advisory Committee Application 1395, February, 2016.

AWAKE CRANIOTOMY

Brain surgeons have been doing brain surgery while the patient is awake for decades. Surgeon would want to have the patient awake during their brain surgery for a few different reasons. In GBM and HGG surgery, the primary reason is to avoid causing damage to a critical area of the brain. Usually, the area of concern involves speech or an area critical for movement. By having the patient awake during part of the surgery, the patient's speech and motor function can be tested. If the patient's speech or motor function gets worse during the surgery, then the surgeon knows that if they continue, they may cause a permanent problem. This would be a reason for the surgeon to stop the surgery to ensure the patient doesn't suffer a major disabling complication.

Most GBM and HGG surgery does not require the patient to be awake. Only when the tumor is located near one of these very important areas would this be appropriate to consider. Not every brain surgeon is comfortable doing awake surgery and may not offer it as part of their practice. In addition, not every anesthesiologist (the doctor who keeps the patient asleep during surgery) is comfortable providing the type of anesthesia that makes awake brain surgery safe and possible.

WHAT TO EXPECT WITH SURGERY

Brain surgery carries with it a certain mystery, fear, and humor in popular culture, but if you're the patient, it all kind of gets reduced to fear. So what will the day of surgery and the days after surgery look and feel like? Understanding that each patient is different and that not all experiences are exactly the same, I will try to describe in general terms what to expect.

DAY OF SURGERY

You may already be in the hospital at this point because of a problem that caused you to go to the emergency room, or you may have been scheduled ahead of time and are showing up from home. Either way, you underwent some blood and urine tests to make sure you're ready and can safely undergo surgery. You washed your hair, face, and neck with a special antibacterial soap a few hours ago. You'll be taken to a preop holding area and shortly after that into the operating room. At some point during this process, there's a good chance your hair is going to need to be cut. Dealing with hair for brain surgery is a science as well as an art for your surgeon. My nurse practitioner actually has a hair salon in his house and takes tremendous pride in how we create the best possible solutions for our patients and their hair.

In general, we try to keep the patient's hair looking as presentable as possible after surgery. What your hair looks like after surgery depends on what your hairstyle was before, where your tumor is, and what your attitude is about your hair. I've done huge brain surgeries to remove large tumors and not removed one strand of hair, and I've also had patients tell me, "Just shave it all off! I don't care."

I would not recommend that you cut your own hair before surgery thinking you're going to help the situation. I had one patient with a very large, very involved, very Irish family who was scheduled to have brain surgery the Monday after St. Patrick's Day. In some sort of spur-of-the-moment, impulsive act of humor while coping with a difficult situation, the entire family shaved all their hair off and painted their heads green. Of course, the patient did this, too, and they all showed up at the hospital the next day with their green heads. Unfortunately, the surgery had to be delayed because we couldn't get the dye off her scalp!

If your appearance is important to you, there's nothing wrong with asking your surgeon what his plan is for your hair. Your surgeon wants you to be happy, and you might be surprised how negotiable this issue is.

Surgery can take thirty minutes or fifteen hours. The length is dependent on way too many factors to discuss in this book. But your surgeon should be able to give you and your family a rough idea of how long they can expect to wait.

AFTER SURGERY

After surgery, you'll be sent to a recovery room that is for all types of patients who are also waking up from anesthesia after all types of surgery. You can expect to be there about an hour, and then you'll likely be sent to the intensive care unit, or ICU. You're not in the ICU because you're a critically ill or unstable patient. You're in the ICU because after brain surgery you may require special medications, special nursing care, and frequent nursing checks, and that can only be done in the ICU. The nurses taking care of you have likely been specially trained to care for brain surgery patients. Most patients only spend a day or two in the ICU and are then moved to a regular floor in the hospital for patients recovering from surgery or dealing with neurologic problems.

Pain after brain surgery is thankfully not a huge problem for most patients. Use of over-the-counter pain medication such as acetaminophen or mild narcotic pain medication is usually all that's needed to keep you comfortable.

At this point, you should be eating, talking, going to the bathroom, and working with a physical, occupational, or speech therapist. After a couple more days on the regular floor, if you pass the evaluations by the therapists, then you may be discharged home in the care of your family. If you are working through a physical or cognitive disability after surgery, then you may require a longer stay or a transfer to a rehabilitation facility or floor until you've improved enough to go home.

Once you're home, you're going to rest. I like to tell patients, "Act like every day is Sunday." Now is not the time to catch up on all the work and to-do lists you've been neglecting while getting your brain surgery. You're not going to do any strenuous activity, no bending or lifting. Your surgeon will want you up and moving but nothing considered vigorous exercise. You can get out of the house for short, easy trips, such as going to church or visiting friends if you feel well enough. You will likely *not* be allowed to *drive*.

You'll follow up with your surgeon in two or three weeks, when these restrictions will start to be reviewed and loosened.

TAKEAWAYS:

- Medical studies have shown that brain surgery that safely removes most of the tumor is the most effective treatment for keeping GBM under control.

- Taking a biopsy to diagnose the tumor may be the first step before a larger surgery to remove the tumor.

- Surgeons have a variety of tools and technologies available to make GBM removal safe and effective for the majority of patients.

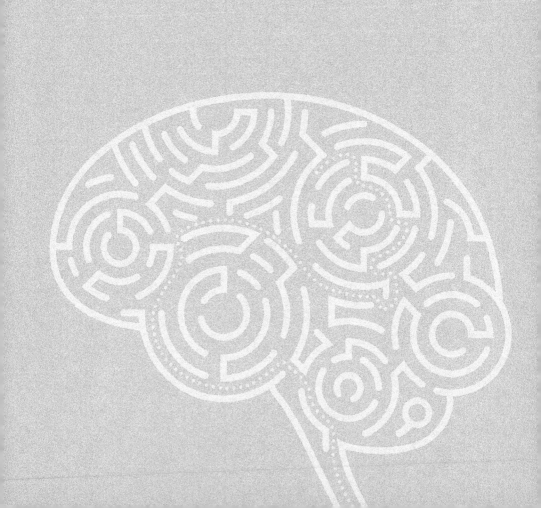

CHAPTER 6

CHEMOTHERAPY AND OTHER MEDICATIONS

Is chemotherapy necessary to treat GBM?

What side effects from chemotherapy can I expect?

Am I going to be on dozens of medications?

About a week after surgery, I received Kevin's pathology report. It was delayed a few days while we waited to receive the complete molecular and genetic information about the tumor from one of the universities that we work with. The final diagnosis was GBM, exactly what I was afraid of.

We called Kevin and brought him and Julie and their parents into the office to talk about the pathology report and what the diagnosis of GBM meant for them.

These are always very emotional meetings, and we try to make sure there is family and/or friend support at this meeting. What makes this meeting challenging is the need to break the difficult news to the patient that they have cancer, but we still need to have a meaningful conversation about the next steps and start planning the treatment. Often after you tell the patient about their diagnosis, they will lose focus and tune out the rest of the conversation as they start to cope with this difficult news. That's why it's important to go to this and all your medical appointments with someone else who can remain emotionally detached, listen, process information, ask questions, and take notes.

Kevin met with our medical oncologist a few days later to plan his chemotherapy treatments.

CHEMOTHERAPY

The dictionary definition for the word *chemotherapy* is any therapeutic use of a chemical (medication) to treat disease. For most people, however, the word *chemotherapy* is associated with the treatment of cancer. This chapter will provide information on the standard chemotherapy medications that are part of treatment for a GBM or HGG.

For many people, the thought of chemotherapy is almost as scary as surgery. Images of hair loss, nausea, vomiting, fatigue, IVs, and spending hours in a chemotherapy center getting medication come to mind.

There are *many* different categories of chemotherapy, and all target different types of cancer in different ways. Each category also has its own side effects. Some chemotherapy regimens are strong and have difficult side effects while others are as easy as taking a daily vitamin. Chemotherapies have changed over the years and now have fewer side effects and are easier to administer. There are now many medications that can manage side effects, should you develop any.

THE BLOOD-BRAIN BARRIER

Chemotherapy for any type of cancer in the brain poses some unique challenges. In order for chemotherapy to work, it must get into your bloodstream. Once in your bloodstream, the medication is circulated in the body until it reaches its targeted cancer cell. The challenge with brain cancer is that even though the brain gets plenty of blood flow, the chemotherapy can't easily reach the cancer cells in the brain.

Most medications have difficulty getting into the brain because the brain has a special ability, similar to a filter, to protect itself, and this stops medications and other substances from getting into the brain. This ability is called the *blood-brain barrier*. Your brain is like a very exclusive club; it's very selective and careful about who and what it lets in. The "doorman" to the club is the blood-brain barrier. If the doorman doesn't recognize you or thinks you're going to be a problem, he won't let you into the club. Most chemotherapy and medications that kill cancers can't get past the doorman in the brain. Chemotherapy for GBM and HGG is designed with the understanding that it has to get past the doorman.

FIRST-LINE CHEMOTHERAPY

The first line of chemotherapy for GBM and HGG is called temozolomide, sold under the brand name Temodar. Temozolomide has been available for GBM and HGG since 2005.

Temozolomide is a pill. There is no IV port and no daily visits to a cancer center. Temozolomide is a type of chemotherapy called *cytotoxic,* meaning its job is to find and kill cancer cells. Specifically, temozolomide alters the

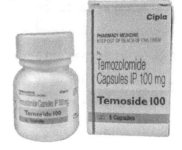

tumor cell's DNA, causing breaks in the DNA chain so the tumor cell cannot divide. Temozolomide is swallowed as a pill, is absorbed by your intestines, and gets into your bloodstream, where it travels to your brain. Once in your bloodstream, it has the ability to cross the blood-brain barrier in sufficient amounts to kill GBM and HGG cells.

Temozolomide is started at the same time as radiation treatment, and it is initially taken once a day for about four to six weeks. Once the radiation treatments are finished, temozolomide is prescribed as one pill a day for five days of every twenty-eight days. If the patient is doing well, temozolomide is typically given for a year, then stopped.

Most people who take temozolomide have little or no side effects. The most common are nausea and vomiting and a low blood cell count. Rarely, there is a loss of appetite, constipation or diarrhea, skin rash, tiredness, weakness, mouth sores, headache, and temporary hair loss. Liver problems can also occur. While taking temozolomide, you will meet with your oncologist on a regular basis, usually monthly, to see how you're tolerating the chemotherapy. The oncologist will also do routine blood work to monitor for any side effects.

Bevacizumab, brand name Avastin, is a chemotherapy medication also approved by the Food and Drug Administration (FDA) for treatment of GBM and HGG. Bevacizumab is considered a second-line chemotherapy, meaning it is usually used only after a GBM or HGG has recurred following a regimen of temozolomide or if the patient cannot take or tolerate temozolomide. Bevacizumab is given as an intravenous infusion every two weeks. Bevacizumab works by preventing the tumor from growing new blood vessels. This has the effect of slowing growth or causing the tumor to become starved of oxygen and blood. A few of the most frequent side effects of bevacizumab are bloody nose, headache, hypertension, a runny nose, protein in the urine, altered taste, and dry skin. Bevacizumab may be combined with a second chemotherapy called lomustine, or CCNU.

Lomustine works by interfering with the tumor's DNA and slowing its growth. Lomustine is given orally in six- to eight-week intervals. It works by altering the tumor's DNA to prevent the tumor from growing. More of a response is seen in tumors that exhibit the MGMT promoter-methylated gene. Common side effects include nausea and vomiting, to the extent that this medication is often given with an additional medication to control those reactions. Myelosuppression, a decrease in the production of some types of blood cells, particularly white blood cells that fight infection and platelets that clot blood, also can occur. While on lomustine, your blood counts have to be watched closely, and the medication may be stopped for a period of time if your blood counts drop too low.

Some oncologists will give lomustine and bevacizumab chemotherapies either alone or together. Whether these two chemotherapies are given alone or in combination, at the moment the scientific data is not conclusive as to how effective they are. Several studies suggest that these chemotherapies, used either alone or in combination, will increase what is called *progression-free survival*, or PFS. PFS means that proof of tumor growth or progression, usually on MRI, is delayed with these medications. That sounds positive, and PFS probably improves the quality of life in many patients. But in most studies these chemotherapies, either alone or in combination, do *not* show an increase in the overall length of survival of the patient.

INTRATUMORAL CHEMOTHERAPY

Gliadel is a product that has a chemotherapy called carmustine, brand name BICNU, which is infused into a small wafer about the size of a nickel. After the tumor has been removed, the wafers are surgically implanted into the brain in the area where the tumor was removed. Carmustine wafers are approved to be used in newly diagnosed GBM and HGG as well as GBM and HGG that has recurred. Once in your brain, the wafer slowly dissolves and releases the chemotherapy into the surrounding brain tissue. The chemotherapy only penetrates a few centimeters into the surrounding tissue, but the idea is that the chemotherapy is killing microscopic cancer cells that could not be removed with surgery.

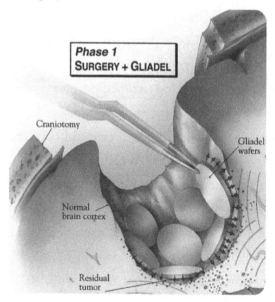

Carmustine wafers can have the side effect of brain swelling, resulting in new neurologic problems. They are also associated with some wound-healing problems. Not all cancer centers that treat GBM will offer carmustine wafers. While the medical data for the wafers does show a survival benefit, it is limited. Some cancer specialists feel the risks of a complication are difficult to justify given the limited benefit to the patient.

GENETIC AND MOLECULAR MARKERS

Most, if not all, GBM/HGG tumors are now tested for a variety of different genetic and molecular traits. You will hear the terms *methylation, gene deletion, wild type,* and *IDH.* These are examples of different biochemical markers that may be found in GBM tissue. This testing is done to further subclassify the tumor. GBM tumors that exhibit methylation of the MGMT promoter gene, 1p19q codeletion, or IDH 1 or 2 mutation may have a better response rate to chemo and radiation and thus may have a better prognosis. Right now, the exact value of these biomarkers is still being studied and may not be used to guide treatment. They do, however, play an important role in research and the development of new and hopefully more effective treatments.

If your GBM/HGG continues to show growth or progression even after surgery, temozolomide, bevacizumab, and lomustine, then it would be important to consider experimental treatments, also called clinical trials, as the next step. More information about experimental trials will be discussed in chapter 11.

In addition to chemotherapy, there are a few other medications that will be part of your treatment at various stages.

STEROIDS

GBM and HGG tumors always cause the normal brain around the tumor to react. This inflammation and edema are the response of the normal brain tissue to the tumor tissue. The edema or swelling is often the cause of many of the symptoms people have from the tumor. Dexamethasone, brand name Decadron, is a steroid that can be given intravenously or as a pill. Decadron given for several days does a very good job of reducing the swelling and edema in the brain, and patients will usually feel better as the symptoms temporarily improve.

After surgery it is very common to go home with a prescription for dexamethasone and instructions from your doctor to take it for several days. When it is time for you to stop taking dexamethasone, the doctor will tell you to decrease the dose slowly over several days. *Never* stop this medicine all at once.

Dexamethasone may be restarted at various times. Brain swelling and edema can return if the tumor grows or returns. Radiation can also cause brain edema or swelling several weeks later.

Many people are bothered by the idea of being on steroids because of potential side effects. However, most of the more serious side effects of steroids are only seen with very long-term use of the medications. Short-term use of ten to fourteen days is not associated with significant side effects in most patients.

SEIZURE MEDICATION

Antiseizure medications may also be part of your treatment. Certainly, if you actually have a seizure, then antiseizure medications will be necessary to control the seizures and may be a long-term addition to your treatment. It is also very common to temporarily put a patient on an antiseizure medication before and after surgery to prevent a seizure during the postoperative time.

Several different types of antiseizure medications exist. Which medication you are placed on is up to the preference of your doctors, but the most common antiseizure medication given during the time of initial diagnosis and surgery is levetiracetam, brand name Keppra. Other medications that might be used include lacosamide (Vimpat), phenytoin (Dilantin), and lamotrigine (Lamictal), among others. All these medications come with advantages, disadvantages, and side effects. A discussion of the effects of antiseizure medications is beyond the scope of this book. You should be sure to discuss them with your treatment team if they are going to be a long-term part of your treatment.

TAKEAWAYS:

- Medical studies have shown that chemotherapy is an effective and essential part of controlling GBM and HGG.

- The initial chemotherapy for GBM and HGG, temozolomide, is taken as a pill and is generally well tolerated, with most patients having mild or no side effects.

- GBM and HGG patients may require a few different medications during their treatment course to manage symptoms from the tumor or side effects from treatments.

CHAPTER 7

RADIATION THERAPY

Is radiation necessary to treat GBM?

What side effects from radiation can I expect?

The third component of GBM and HGG treatment, along with surgery and chemotherapy, is radiation therapy. Radiation therapy has been around since the 1950s and has evolved over the decades to become a safe and effective tool in treating many types of cancer, including GBM and HGG. Radiation cancer specialists use high-energy X-ray techniques to treat tumors. Several different types and techniques of radiation treatment are used to treat both benign and cancerous brain tumors. These radiation treatments all have different roles and uses. Let's try to understand how radiation is used in GBM and HGG.

HOW RADIATION WORKS AGAINST CANCER CELLS

Radiation therapy targets the brain tumor with high-energy photons. A photon is an invisible particle with a tremendous amount of energy, released by certain radioactive substances. When a high-energy photon interacts with tissues of the body, it causes damage to cells. Radiation damages a cell in two basic ways. The first is by damaging the DNA of the cell so that it cannot reproduce, divide, or function. The second is by damaging the sensitive tissues of the blood vessels that supply the cell. When the cell damaged by the radiation is part of a tumor, it causes the tumor tissue to stop growing and die.

RADIATION TREATMENT FOR GBM/HGG

Rapidly dividing cancer cells such as GBM and HGG can be very sensitive to radiation treatments. The goal of radiation therapy is to deliver radiation to the tumor while sparing the normal, healthy tissue surrounding the tumor. The worry is that despite more precise delivery methods, radiation can "scatter" and might affect normal healthy cells as well as cancer cells. Radiation treatment for GBM and HGG occurs after surgery and is done with the first cycle of temozolomide. Radiation and chemotherapy typically start two to four weeks after surgery to allow the surgical wound to heal.

THE GOAL OF RADIATION THERAPY IS TO DELIVER RADIATION TO THE TUMOR WHILE SPARING THE NORMAL, HEALTHY TISSUE SURROUNDING THE TUMOR.

Radiation treatments are extensive. Intensity-modulated radiation therapy (IMRT) is the standard type of radiation treatment for GBM and HGG. The treatment plan is tailored for each patient depending on where the tumor is, how large it is, what area involved, and whether any tumor is still seen on MRI after surgery. These treatments will be given five days a week, usually for a duration of six weeks. Radiation treatments are not uncomfortable, but most patients report fatigue as the most frequent side effect.

TYPES OF RADIATION TREATMENTS

There are several other types of radiation treatments used for brain tumors, but IMRT has been proven to be most effective at controlling GBM and HGG. The other types of radiation that you may hear about include Gamma Knife; stereotactic radiotherapy, or SRS; CyberKnife; or ZAP. These are all very similar technologies and may sound much more appealing than IMRT because they are very precise and can treat a brain tumor in usually one to three patient visits instead of six weeks. Unfortunately, several research studies have shown that while these precise, short-duration treatments are very effective for treating *metastatic cancer* that has spread to the brain (i.e., lung cancer, colon cancer, etc.), they are not as effective at treating GBM and HGG. This is because GBM/HGG spreads to the surrounding brain tissue with very small, microscopic areas of cancer that cannot be seen on an MRI. IMRT is designed to target the area of the tumor seen on MRI plus a generous margin of brain surrounding the tumor in an effort to treat these unseen and very small areas of GBM.

POSSIBLE SIDE EFFECTS OF RADIATION

The side effects of the radiation treatment are not common but can include brain swelling and edema, which can result in headache, seizure, nausea, vomiting, or new neurologic problems. As the tumor cells die, the surrounding brain can react to the "injured" tumor with swelling and edema. As the radiation effect takes place, the tumor undergoes a process called *necrosis*. Necrosis is the death of tumor cells. Necrosis means the radiation treatment is working and destroying the tumor tissue. Radiation necrosis can also cause brain swelling and mimic growth of the tumor. On an MRI, that swelling and radiation effect may give the appearance of tumor growth or progression. This is called *pseudoprogression*, or false progression.

Special MRI techniques exist that can help doctors tell the difference between pseudoprogression from radiation and actual tumor growth. MR spectroscopy and MR perfusion are specific types of MRI used to try to distinguish between pseudoprogression and actual tumor growth.

In rare circumstances, a biopsy of the area or repeat surgery is needed to decide if the tumor has recurred or to treat symptoms from radiation necrosis.

For most GBM and HGG patients, one course of IMRT is all the radiation that will be needed. Even if the tumor returns or grows, more radiation is usually not an option. The maximum amount of effective radiation is usually given in the initial six-week course of treatment, and more radiation has not been proven to be helpful.

There may be rare situations where more or a different radiation course will be tried for recurrent GBM/HGG when there are no other treatment options for the patient. This is when the short-duration precision radiation mentioned earlier (Gamma Knife, CyberKnife, ZAP) may be considered. That would not be considered usual care and is outside the NCCN Guidelines.

GAMMATILE THERAPY

GammaTile therapy is a type of radiation treatment where radiation "seeds" are implanted into the surgical cavity after the tumor is removed.

This treatment is FDA approved for all malignant brain tumors, including GBM and HGG.

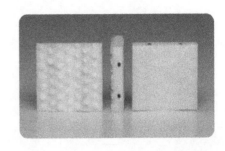

GammaTile treatment is a sliver of radioactive cesium inside a small square of fibrous backing that is implanted into the cavity after the tumor is removed. The cesium then releases radiation into the surrounding brain to further treat cancerous GBM cells. Currently, GammaTile is not part of the NCCN Guidelines for GBM and HGG and has not been proven to be more effective than standard IMRT radiation for GBM and HGG. But for some patients, especially those who have already received the maximum amount of IMRT radiation, GammaTile may be a useful addition to treatment. The data for GammaTile use with regard to GBM and HGG is very preliminary, but early results show it to be safe with very few side effects and effective at improving overall survival.

TAKEAWAYS:

- Medical studies have shown that IMRT radiation is an important and effective part of GBM treatment.

- Radiation is usually low risk and well tolerated, with few side effects.

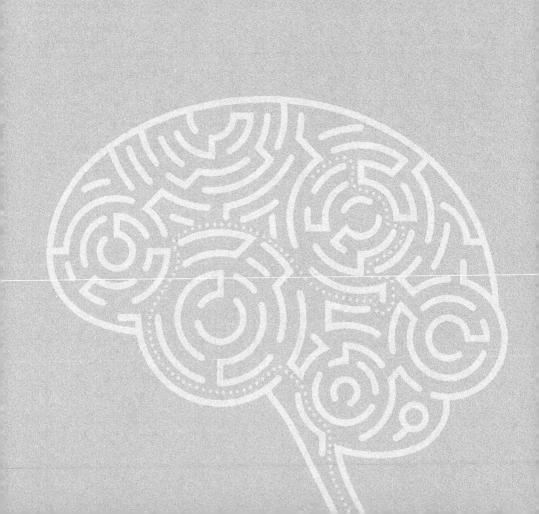

CHAPTER 8

NEUROLOGIC DISABILITIES AND COPING WITH THEM

● ●

> What kind of neurologic problems can happen with a brain tumor?
>
> Are neurologic problems seen with a brain tumor or after surgery permanent?

My father, an attorney and judge in our hometown, was well known among the legal community. I was talking to him on the phone one day when I was in residency training, and he told me an awful story about a good friend of his who was the local chief of police. This friend, a very respected, distinguished police officer, had just been arrested for shoplifting! Of course, this completely baffled the legal community, family, and friends, who struggled to understand this behavior.

As his criminal case for shoplifting worked its way through the courts, he was caught stealing again, this time from a gas station! The cause of his behavior was revealed when he had a massive seizure, which prompted his doctors to scan his brain, only to find a massive tumor occupying the entire front of his brain! The tumor eventually was diagnosed as a GBM.

When I heard the result of his brain scan, it all became very clear. His shoplifting was easily explained by the loss of function of the part of his brain called the frontal lobes. The good news was that the poor judge's reputation was restored, and he didn't go to jail. The bad news was that this was only because he had a brain tumor.

There is a lot about the brain that we still don't understand, but we do have a working understanding about certain important functions and their location in the brain. Tumors that occur in certain areas of the brain will result in a predictable sign or symptom in the patient. In the case of my father's colleague, the behavior and the seizure were the results of a tumor located in the frontal lobe of the brain.

TUMORS THAT OCCUR IN CERTAIN AREAS OF THE BRAIN WILL RESULT IN A PREDICTABLE SIGN OR SYMPTOM IN THE PATIENT.

It's important to understand that just because a tumor is in one of the locations described in this chapter, it doesn't mean the patient will have all or even some of the neurological problems mentioned. Symptoms can range from mild, such as a headache that won't go away, to more serious symptoms such as seizures or speech difficulties.

Let's review a brief anatomy lesson to understand the location of important areas of the brain.

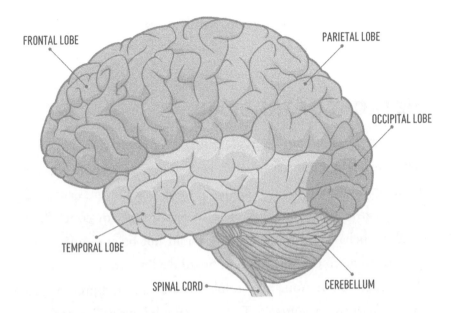

FRONTAL LOBE

PARIETAL LOBE

OCCIPITAL LOBE

TEMPORAL LOBE

SPINAL CORD

CEREBELLUM

LEFT AND RIGHT

Your brain is divided into two halves: left and right. Motor function and sensation *cross over*: the *left* side of your brain is responsible for making your *right* arm and *right* leg move, and vice versa. So, if you are *right handed*, then the *left* half of your brain is particularly important to your daily function. Regarding sensation, the situation is the same: the *left* side of your brain will receive the information from your *right* hand that it's hot when it touches a hot stove.

Language is a bit different. When I refer to language, I'm talking about your ability to speak and your ability to understand when someone else is speaking. For about 90 percent of us, language function is in the *left* half of the brain. A small percentage of people will have language function in the *right* half, though the reason for this is unknown.

So, if you're right handed, like most, it's pretty obvious that the *left* side of your brain is super important to your ability to live a normal life. For most, left-brain problems can be devastating to a person's normal daily function.

THE FRONT OF THE BRAIN

The front halves of your brain are called the *frontal lobes*. You have a left and a right frontal lobe. Frontal lobes are responsible for higher-level thinking and judgment, what is sometimes referred to as *executive functions*. They are also responsible for controlling impulsive behavior. For example, it would not be appropriate for someone to go to the bathroom in broad daylight in the middle of a busy intersection. Your frontal lobes realize this and prevent you from embarrassing yourself. Take our shoplifting policeman: his frontal lobe tumor impaired his judgment and his ability to control the impulse to steal from the gas station.

THE BACK OF THE BRAIN

The back part of your brain is called the *occipital lobes*. You have a left and a right occipital lobe. The most important job of the occipital lobes is vision. Vision also crosses over, meaning your *right* occipital lobe is responsible for the *left* half of your vision in your left eye and the *left* half of vision in your right eye, and vice versa. Problems with one of your occipital lobes will *not* make you completely blind in both eyes, or even in one eye, but you will lose a portion of the vision in each eye.

Often a person may not realize that they have a vision problem until the doctor asks questions like "How many times have you sideswiped a parked car in the last few months?" or "How many times have you hit the side of the garage trying to pull the car in?"

The patient and his family wonder how the doctor could know these things! These are examples of predictable symptoms specific to the area of the brain where the tumor is located.

TEMPORAL AND PARIETAL AREAS

Symptoms of a *temporal lobe* or a *parietal lobe* tumor may be subtle and difficult to detect due to the anatomy and physiology of the brain and its structures. Seizures are often the first neurologic problem experienced with a temporal lobe tumor. Deep temporal tumors can cause short-term memory problems. Left temporal tumors can sometimes cause problems understanding language and speaking. In the parietal lobe, the most obvious problem would be weakness or numbness in one side of the body.

SEIZURE

Any person who has a structural problem in their brain, regardless of the reason (tumor, stroke, trauma), is more susceptible to having a seizure. At its most fundamental level, your brain works by sending electrical/chemical signals back and forth in a controlled manner. In a seizure, these electoral/chemical signals are out of control.

It doesn't matter where your tumor is in the brain; a seizure can come from any part. The first clue that you have a brain tumor of any kind may be a seizure. Seizures can be terrifying for the patient and anyone witnessing it. Fortunately, they are usually short lived (lasting only minutes), and very often the patient recovers quickly. But occasionally a seizure can be prolonged and dangerous.

The first time someone has a seizure, it is probably best to call 9-1-1 and get immediate medical attention. For some patients with

GBM, seizures become a repeated problem. Medication can often be successful in controlling seizures, though sometimes, even when taking several seizure medications, repeat seizures can still be an issue for some patients. Your doctors may refer you to a neurologist who specializes in seizures to help treat this problem.

From a lifestyle / quality of life perspective, seizures can be a big problem. Safety is always a concern when a person has poorly controlled seizures. Because of the risk of injury, a person who has frequent seizures should not be left alone for prolonged periods of time. If the person lives alone, having a seizure condition can be a big concern. Electronic monitoring devices that can summon help may be useful should a person fall or feel a seizure starting.

Driving a car, cooking, swimming, boating, climbing—these are just a few of the safety risks for those who have seizures.

Taking away a person's driving privileges can "add insult to injury." On top of coping with a diagnosis of GBM or HGG, dealing with chemo and radiation, and recovering from surgery, plus a million other things, the doctors may say that the patient cannot drive. Driving any motorized vehicle is a major safety concern for patients with seizures. A seizure while driving can cause a serious accident that results in injury to the person having the seizure as well as to others. Each state has different laws regarding *if and under what conditions* a person who has seizures can drive. But the ultimate responsibility is the patient's and their family's. Safety, safety, safety.

It is important to repeat that just because a tumor is in one of the locations described in this chapter, it doesn't mean the patient will have all, or even some, of the neurologic problems mentioned.

COPING WITH A NEUROLOGIC PROBLEM

Since the diagnosis of GBM *may* come with certain neurologic struggles, it is important to understand how to cope with them. Often these problems are temporary, but occasionally they can be permanent.

We've already touched on the dangers of driving in the context of a seizure, but driving can also be an issue when other neurologic problems are present. If you are right handed and have weakness or coordination problems with your right hand or leg, the ability to drive safely may be a challenge. If vision is affected by an occipital lobe tumor, safe driving can be a struggle. A frontal lobe tumor can cause impaired judgment, compromised decision-making, and delayed reaction time, all of which can impact driving safely.

Returning to work after surgery or after diagnosis of GBM or HGG can be a complicated decision for the patient and family. For some people, returning to work will be difficult or not an option because of a disability. And yet, many will get through the initial surgery and treatment with little difficulty, making returning to work an option. But many people will take the diagnosis of GBM/HGG as an opportunity to not return to work and instead to focus on their health and spending time with loved ones.

Other disabilities such as arm and leg weakness, balance problems, and/or impaired memory, cognitive function, and judgment can all impact the safety and quality of a person's life. Walkers, canes, and wheelchairs may temporarily or permanently become part of the person's life. Neurologic disabilities can also affect the home as well as relationships with friends and family. Ramps may need to be built, doors widened to accommodate wheelchairs, and bathrooms modified. Personality changes due to the location of the GBM may be seen and may affect relationships. The patient may become impulsive, depressed, and in denial of their disability, may attempt unsafe activities, and may require close supervision.

Physical, occupational, speech, memory, and cognitive therapies can all be very helpful to address, adjust to, and potentially overcome these challenges and accelerate the patient's recovery. These services are often provided within a day of surgery while recovering in the hospital. Therapy can continue on an outpatient basis with the therapist going to the home or at an outpatient physical therapy location. When necessary, therapy can continue at an inpatient rehabilitation facility.

The diagnosis of GBM or HGG almost always starts with some sort of neurologic problem or disability. This neurologic problem may be temporary and improve as the patient moves through treatment, or it may become permanent and require minor or major adjustments to the life of the patient and their friends and family. On top of coping with a neurologic problem, anyone who has received a cancer diagnosis must cope with the inevitable feelings of anxiety, fatigue, and depression. Support groups for both family and the patient exist for GBM, HGG, brain tumors in general and for anyone who is learning to cope with a new neurologic problem.

TAKEAWAYS:

- The diagnosis of GBM and HGG will almost always start with some sort of neurologic problem.

- Neurologic problems from a brain tumor can widely vary from mild headache to significant speech problems or physical disabilities.

- Neurologic problems from GBM and HGG very often are temporary or significantly improve with treatment. In some cases, neurologic problems from GBM and HGG may be permanent, but resources are available to patients and families to cope with and overcome these issues.

CHAPTER 9

RECURRENCE

· ·

> How will I know if the tumor has recurred or progressed?
>
> What steps are taken if there is tumor recurrence or progression?

Kevin got through a very successful surgery with no neurologic problems. We discussed his pathology results, got him through six weeks of radiation, and had him start cycling on and off temozolomide every month. He eventually returned to work.

He came in every three months for an MRI of his brain with contrast, and the daily rhythm of his life returned to normal.

He did a total of twelve cycles of temozolomide, lasting a little over a year from the time he was first diagnosed. About four months after stopping the temozolomide, his MRI started to show a small area of change right next to his original surgery. This area enhanced with contrast was clearly not seen in his earlier imaging. The area I was concerned about was small, about the size of a large grape, and Kevin was feeling well, having no symptoms or neurologic problems.

I met with Kevin's oncologist, radiation oncologist, and radiologist to review the latest MRI. I also sent his images to a second comprehensive cancer center for review. We all agreed this was most likely new growth or a recurrence of his GBM.

We brought Kevin and his family into the office to talk about the new MRI findings and outline his next treatment options. Kevin's tumor was still in the left front of his brain and looked like it could be removed with a second surgery with an acceptable amount of risk. This, coupled with the fact that Kevin was otherwise completely healthy and functioning normally, made the decision to return to surgery easy.

Once we got Kevin through his second surgery, the next step would be to discuss what "second-line chemotherapy" would look like. In Kevin's case, the area of the brain in which the new tumor was found had already received the maximum amount of radiation, so more radiation treatments were not an option.

Kevin and his wife were, of course, disappointed with the news that the tumor had recurred, but they were not surprised. They have always had a realistic understanding of what GBM means and that cures are rare.

With our plan agreed upon among the patient, his family, and his doctors, we took him back to surgery.

THINGS TO CONSIDER WHEN THE TUMOR RECURS

There are long-term GBM/HGG patients without a recurrence in the world, but unfortunately, for almost every person who receives the diagnosis, even after perfect surgery, world-class care, and the best treatment that medicine has to offer, the tumor will almost always come back.

Your journey so far has been a brain tumor was discovered, surgery was performed, the GBM or HGG diagnosis was made, you finished radiation treatments, you've been on and off temozolomide, you've recovered, and your life has returned to near normal. Your three-month follow-up appointment is coming up shortly. You have an MRI and go to your appointment to meet with the oncologist or neurosurgeon. They tell you they see some changes on your MRI. Your heart sinks. What happens next?

The first thing that you and your doctor want is an accurate interpretation of the MRI. Are we looking at true tumor progression and growth? Or are we looking at pseudoprogression or radiation damage? Or is something else occurring, such as an infection or an abscess? Sometimes the answers to these questions are straightforward. For example, if a new finding on the MRI looks like a tumor, is surrounded by edema and swelling, enhances, and is located far from the original tumor, then there's a good chance the GBM or HGG has returned or progressed.

However, if the new finding on MRI is right next to where the previous tumor was, has fuzzy or poorly defined edges, and is in the area that was treated with radiation, then *maybe* it's not tumor recurrence. *Maybe* this is radiation damage showing up several weeks or months later, or *maybe* it's the beginning of a postsurgical infection or abscess.

This is when an MR perfusion scan or MR spectroscopy scan (discussed in chapter 7) may be helpful. These tests may help your treatment team distinguish between true tumor recurrence and something that is imitating tumor recurrence.

Often when changes in the MRI occur, the MRI images will be presented to the tumor board and the entire treatment team for collective discussion. They can pool their experience and knowledge to make recommendations for next steps in your care.

If the MRI images are not conclusive and no further information can be gathered from one of the specialized MRI techniques, then surgery may be recommended for a definitive answer. The other option that the treatment team may recommend is to just watch the changes and repeat the MRI in a few weeks. If the images are conclusive for tumor recurrence, then your treatment team will recommend additional treatments for you to consider.

TREATMENT OPTIONS FOR A RECURRENCE

Once the treatment team is convinced that you have recurrence or progression of the tumor, either by surgical biopsy result or convincing MRI changes, they will discuss what the treatment options are at this point.

Treatment decisions and options are not as straightforward when dealing with a recurrence compared to when you were first diagnosed. First and foremost, the condition of the patient must be assessed. Very often the Karnofsky Performance Scale discussed in chapter 4 will be used to assess the overall function of the patient.

TREATMENT DECISIONS AND OPTIONS ARE NOT AS STRAIGHTFORWARD WHEN DEALING WITH A RECURRENCE COMPARED TO WHEN YOU WERE FIRST DIAGNOSED.

Some people, like Kevin, sail through the initial surgery, radiation, and chemo and are full of energy, moving ahead in life full speed without interruption. Other people suffer from seizures, are disabled in some way from the original tumor, are dependent on their family for their basic care, or have side effects from the chemotherapy. The condition of the patient at the time of recurrence will play an important role in what treatment options are reasonable to pursue.

MORE SURGERY

Because surgery is often the most effective weapon we have to treat GBM and HGG, the first question asked at the time of recurrence is "Can the recurrent tumor be removed with surgery?" For the answer to be yes, three issues must be considered:

1. Is the patient in good enough shape to get through another brain surgery?

2. Is the tumor in a location that can be safely operated on with reasonable risk?

3. Can the area of recurrence be totally removed?

If the answer to any of these conditions is no, then more surgery *may not* be the best option.

An additional consideration is whether removing all or a significant portion of the recurrent tumor will improve the quality of life for the patient, even though it may not impact the patient's overall survival.

MORE CHEMOTHERAPY

In the world of cancer treatment, a second course of chemotherapy is known as *second-line chemotherapy*. It's called second line because it's not been proven to be as effective as the first recommended type of chemotherapy. Which isn't to say it's *not* effective; it's just not *as* effective. Patients and families need to understand that the scientific evidence for second-line therapy for GBM is not as conclusive compared to first-line treatment. If a GBM or HGG recurs after treatment with first-line temozolomide, the NCCN Guidelines for second-line chemotherapy for GBM/HGG include medications called bevacizumab (Avastin) and lomustine.

Lomustine is given orally in six- to eight-week intervals. It works by altering the tumor's DNA to prevent the tumor from growing. More of a response is seen in tumors that exhibit the MGMT pro-moter-methylated gene. Common side effects include nausea and vomiting, to the extent that this medication is often given with an additional medication to control those side effects. Myelosuppression, a decrease in the production of some types of blood cells, particularly white blood cells that fight infection and platelets that clot blood, can occur. While you are on lomustine, your blood counts must be watched closely, and the medication may be stopped for a period of time if your blood counts drop too low.

Bevacizumab is given as an intravenous infusion every two weeks. It works by a different mechanism from other chemotherapies. Instead of working on the tumor cell DNA like temozolomide and lomustine, it works to shut down the blood supply to the tumor so it cannot grow. The side effects of bevacizumab involve bleeding and blood clotting. Complications can include bleeding in the brain, stroke, and blood clots in the legs or lungs. Also, it may be important to know that surgery of any kind cannot be done while on bevacizumab—it must be stopped for up to four weeks before surgery can be safely performed due to the risk of bleeding. This means that surgery for recurrent GBM must be done *before* you start bevacizumab chemotherapy.

Some oncologists will give these chemotherapies alone or together. The scientific data is not conclusive as to whether these two chemotherapies are best given alone or in combination. Several studies suggest that these chemotherapies either alone or in combination will increase what is called *progression-free survival,* or PFS. PFS means that proof of tumor growth or progression, usually on MRI, is delayed with these medications. That sounds positive, and PFS probably improves the quality of life in many patients. But in most studies, these chemotherapies, either alone or in combination, do *not* show an increase in the overall survival of the patient.

Gliadel wafers (discussed in chapter 6) can also be implanted into the tumor area for a recurrence and have shown a limited benefit to survival in the setting of GBM or HGG recurrence.

Some patients may have the option of becoming involved in an experimental clinical trial at the time of their recurrence.

MORE RADIATION

As we discussed in chapter 7, after your initial treatment with IMRT, more radiation treatments are rarely an option. However, if surgery cannot be done for a recurrence, often additional radiation treatments are considered. A second course of radiation is usually one of the stereotactic radiation techniques discussed in chapter 7 (Gamma Knife, CyberKnife, ZAP). While there is no data to support a survival benefit, it may reduce the need for steroids and has a very low risk of any side effects.

Recurrence of GBM after initial treatment is news that patients and families don't want to hear. Decision-making and understanding your options with GBM recurrence can become complicated with new testing, less-than-certain results, and less concrete treatment options. It is important to stay focused on what your treatment team is recommending and the options that are available to you to navigate the best path forward. But it is also important to remember that for almost every patient, several more treatments are available that are scientifically proven to be safe and effective if your GBM recurs.

TAKEAWAYS:

- The first sign of tumor recurrence or growth may be a new neurologic problem, but usually changes on an MRI will be the first clue that the tumor has grown or progressed.

- For almost every patient, further treatments are available that have been proven to be effective against GBM and HGG if the tumor grows or recurs.

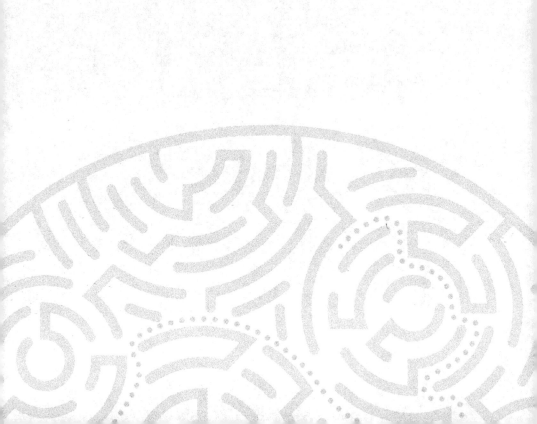

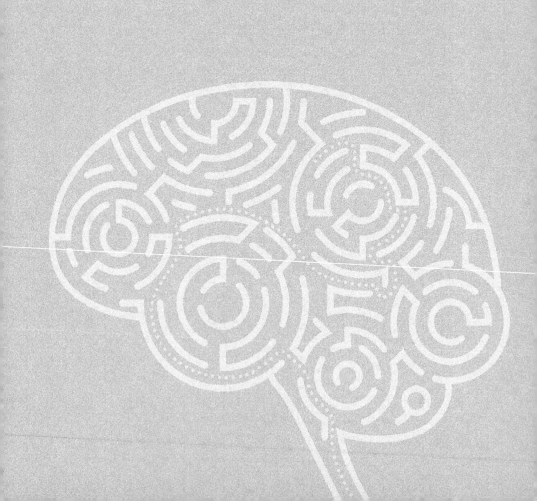

CHAPTER 10

ADDITIONAL TREATMENTS

Are there any proven treatments for GBM besides chemotherapy, radiation, and surgery?

Kevin's second surgery to remove the recurrent tumor was successful, and he recovered well. During that second surgery, I implanted Gliadel chemotherapy wafers into Kevin's brain to further help treat his GBM. Once Kevin healed from his second surgery, his oncologist arranged for him to start bevacizumab and lomustine chemotherapy.

Kevin and his wife were always asking questions and trying to understand everything they could about GBM. They were always interested in any and all possible treatments. When we saw Kevin and his wife in the office, we reviewed his plan and discussed a new nonchemotherapy, nonsurgical treatment for GBM called alternating electrical field therapy, brand name Optune.

We talked about the Optune system and what it involves and how effective it is for GBM. One issue many patients have with Optune is the requirement that you be completely bald to use the system. As you can imagine, for some patients this is a huge issue. Thankfully Kevin started losing his hair in his twenties, and by this point in his life he already was completely bald! He was one of our first patients to use the Optune system.

Besides surgery, chemotherapy, and radiation treatments, other potential treatment options are available for patients. Some of these treatments have been adopted as part of the NCCN Guidelines while other FDA-approved treatments have not.

OPTUNE

Optune is an additional treatment that has been approved by the FDA and was recently included in the NCCN Guidelines for the

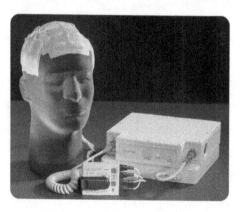

treatment of GBM. Optune is not approved for HGG or other types of gliomas.

The Optune is a device that is worn by the patient and uses alternating electric field therapy to slow the growth or progression of a GBM. The patient wears a device on their head that delivers a programmed electric current through the scalp and skull and into the brain to slow GBM growth. This device is currently approved for the initial diagnosis of GBM and also for GBM that comes back after surgery.

The programmed electrical current created by the Optune device disrupts the tumor cells and their ability to divide and multiply.

To benefit from the device, the patient must shave their head completely about every three days. The patient then attaches several adhesive pads (similar to EKG electrode pads) to their scalp in a specific pattern based on the location of the tumor. The pads are attached to wires on the Optune console. The patient wears or carries the console with them while the treatment is delivered. The console has become smaller and is now the size of a medium purse. To gain the benefit, the device must be worn an average of eighteen hours a day for as long as it is effective. As unpleasant as shaving your head sounds, medical studies have shown a *meaningful improvement in survival* with the use of Optune.

Though the medical data is good and there is evidence of a survival benefit, doctors have difficulty convincing patients to use this device. Shaving your head every three days is a major concern for most people, especially women. From a social perspective, wearing the device in public can be awkward. It's difficult to hide while wearing it. Despite the benefit of improved survival, even with a cancer that has limited survival, many patients have difficulty getting past these issues.

LITT

Conventional surgery remains the best treatment option, but laser interstitial thermal therapy, or LITT, is also an option for certain GBM/HGG patients. LITT may also be called MRI-guided laser ablation and is considered a minimally invasive surgical technique. LITT allows the neurosurgeons to more precisely target and destroy tumor tissue. It is an option for GBM/HGG patients who are not candidates for an extensive brain surgery either because the tumor is in a location in the brain where it is too dangerous to operate or because operating in that part of the brain will cause a significant disability for the patient.

To deliver the LITT treatment, a small hole is drilled in the skull, and a laser probe is carefully inserted into the tumor. The laser is then activated, and the laser energy destroys tumor cells within a certain distance. Anything that can be done to decrease the number of tumor cells is thought to be beneficial in the treatment of GBM and HGG. The laser probe itself is small and can reach tumors in difficult or deep locations. The small size of the laser probe disturbs little or no normal brain tissue, so the risk of damage to the surrounding normal brain is small.

LITT has not been found to be more effective than standard surgery to remove a GBM or HGG. It is worth repeating here that conventional surgery, as described in chapter 5, is still the preferred first treatment option. However, LITT is a reasonable option to consider when the usual surgery is not possible. The research data currently considers LITT an experimental treatment, and it is recommended only when no other surgical options are available.

PARTICLE THERAPY

Particle therapy is a version of radiation therapy that uses subatomic particles to deliver high energy to the tumor instead of the photons used in the other types of radiation treatments that were addressed in chapter 6. The most available example of particle therapy is proton beam therapy.

So what's the difference between a proton and a photon? While there are entire volumes of radiation physics textbooks written on these topics, from the patient's perspective it boils down to a couple of points. All types of radiation therapies are trying to deliver as much energy as possible to destroy tumor cells while limiting the amount of radiation to normal tissue. Proton beam therapy can deliver very high doses of energy to tumors at a specific location and then drop the energy very abruptly to limit the amount of energy given to the normal brain tissue. This sounds like a good option, except the medical studies have not shown any improvement in survival for GBM or HGG with proton beam therapy compared to the more conventional radiation treatments already discussed in chapter 6.

Proton beam treatment also has an additional disadvantage of being very expensive, and most of these machines are only found at major university centers as part of a research program exploring the usefulness of this type of treatment. Proton beam therapy has a very limited role in other kinds of brain tumors, such as rare chordomas, chondrosarcomas, and certain tumors in children. Any use of proton beam therapy in adult GBM or HGG will likely be as part of an experimental treatment.

THE CHALLENGE OF RESEARCHING GBM TREATMENT

The reality of GBM and HGG treatments is that because GBM/HGG is such a unique and rare cancer, it is very difficult to conduct research and prove how effective or ineffective a new treatment might be. For example, the National Cancer Institute lists the thirteen most common cancers in the United States. GBM is so rare that it didn't even make the list of the top thirteen most common. The least common cancer on the list of thirteen was liver cancer, with 42,810 new cases in a year. Compare that to approximately 13,000 new diagnoses of GBM per year.

The relatively small number of patients diagnosed and living with GBM and HGG makes studying the disease and developing treatments challenging. The success and pace of any cancer research comes down to numbers of patients. The more widespread the cancer, the more patients there are to test new treatments on. The more patients enrolled in experimental trials to test new treatments, the easier it is to prove if the treatment is safe and effective.

> **THE RELATIVELY SMALL NUMBER OF PATIENTS DIAGNOSED AND LIVING WITH GBM AND HGG MAKES STUDYING THE DISEASE AND DEVELOPING TREATMENTS CHALLENGING.**

TAKEAWAYS:

- There are certain nonchemotherapy and nonsurgical options for treating GBM and HGG, although their effectiveness varies.

- Be sure to discuss and ask about all treatment options with your treatment team.

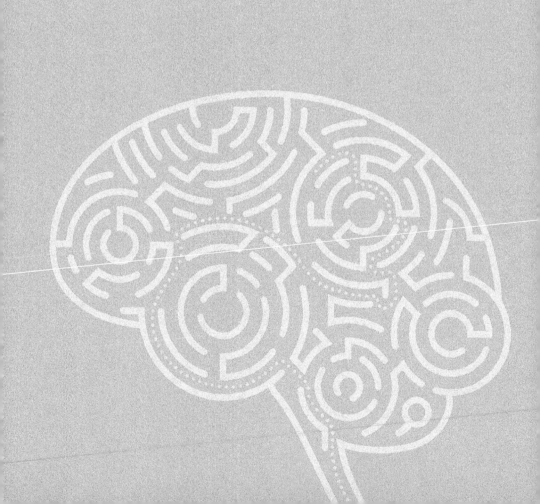

CHAPTER 11

ALTERNATIVE TREATMENTS AND THE ROLE OF DIET, SUPPLEMENTS, AND ATTITUDE

Are there any proven natural or holistic treatments for GBM and HGG?

Why is the medical community not more involved with holistic options?

What kind of diet should I be eating if I have a GBM or HGG?

A physician friend of mine asked me to see his mother, who had been having trouble speaking for the past two weeks. She came to the office, and we examined her. While she could speak words, they were disjointed and made no sense—a speech pattern we call "word salad."

I ordered an MRI of her brain, and she had two large tumors, both close to the part of her brain that controls language. I called my physician friend to give him the MRI results, and he told me a very interesting story that his mother had failed to mention.

His mother had been diagnosed with metastatic lung cancer six years ago but had been doing well and was cancer-free for about the last three years. I asked what treatments she received, and he said she started with the conventional radiation treatment to her lung and then went on an extensive course of chemotherapy. She stopped the chemotherapy after about six months because it made her very sick, and she couldn't see herself continuing with the treatments if they were going to make her so ill.

She began researching alternative treatments for her cancer and found a doctor in Central America that offered "holistic, natural-based" treatments for lung cancer. She flew to Central America several times over the next year and received these holistic treatments while at the same time continuing to follow up with her local oncologist.

For about two years she did very well, with no evidence that her lung cancer was progressing until the brain tumors were found.

Patients often look outside of medicine for ways to cure their cancer. These may be called alternative therapies, holistic treatments, organic treatments, naturopathic remedies, or any number of other names. While there may be some quality-of-life benefit to these alternatives, they are not cancer treatments, and they are outside the boundaries of

THERE IS NO SCIENTIFIC EVIDENCE THAT ALTERNATIVE THERAPIES WILL TREAT OR CURE ANY CANCER OR IMPROVE SURVIVAL.

what medical professionals consider to be the standard of care and practice. In short, there is no scientific evidence that alternative therapies such as vitamins, enemas, herbs, ancient grains, seeds, organic foods, massage therapy, cryotherapy, or naturopathic treatments will treat or cure any cancer or improve survival, but that doesn't necessarily mean they couldn't play a beneficial role in your health and overall well-being.

Some nutritional supplements, herbs, and vitamins may actually interfere with medications prescribed by your doctor, cause liver damage, or interfere with the ability of your blood to clot. At every visit with your doctor, it is important to tell them about any over-the-counter medicine, vitamins, and herbal substances that you are taking. Some alternative options, however, such as good nutrition, massage therapy, and meditation may provide a quality-of-life benefit and help the patient tolerate their treatments better.

WHY THE MEDICAL COMMUNITY MAY BE SKEPTICAL ABOUT ALTERNATIVE TREATMENTS

I can't think of any oncologist who wouldn't embrace and utilize any cancer treatment if they felt it to be safe and it was scientifically proven to be effective for their patients, no matter whether the treatment came from some sort of nutritional-based cure or was engineered by a multimillion-dollar pharmaceutical company. So why is the medical profession so skeptical of the use of alternative treatments?

There are several reasons for this:

1. "AS DOCTORS AND SCIENTISTS, WE'RE TRAINED TO TRUST THE DATA."

Physicians and other health professionals are trained to rely on scientific evidence. The medical profession is distrustful of claims of cures when there is no data-driven scientific proof of effectiveness. Most physicians are concerned about the use of any treatment that is not approved by the FDA or not endorsed by their scientific community.

Often, alternative treatments cite their benefit through what is called *anecdotal evidence*. Anecdotal evidence is when a single example or story is told about one patient or a very small group of patients apparently having a negative or positive effect from something. For example, "My grandma took a shot of whiskey every night before bed, and she never so much as got a cold in her life." This is a lovely anecdote, but it's not scientific proof of the effect of whiskey on preventing the cold. Be wary of any treatment recommended through such anecdotal evidence.

2. "THEY DON'T TEACH US VOODOO IN MEDICAL SCHOOL."

Training for physicians about alternative treatments is almost nonexistent in medical school and fellowship training. If a physician wants to become knowledgeable on these treatments, they usually will have to educate themselves in these areas.

3. "IF I CAN'T GET REIMBURSED FOR IT, THEN I DON'T HAVE TIME TO LEARN IT."

For the most part, medical insurance will only agree to pay for treatments that are approved by the FDA or treatments that are part of a research trial.

4. "IT'S A STRUGGLE TO KEEP UP WITH ALL THE CURRENT DATA AND ADVANCES IN THE SCIENTIFIC AND MEDICAL FIELDS—THERE'S NO TIME TO LEARN ABOUT UNPROVEN TREATMENTS."

Hospitals and physician offices are interested in delivering the most effective and safe treatments. They may want to provide some of the alternative options that do promote wellness, but they are absolutely bound by the limits of their resources, the rules of the FDA, and the lack of insurance reimbursement.

WHY DO PATIENTS SEEK OUT ALTERNATIVE TREATMENTS?

It has become increasingly clear to those who treat cancer patients that the quality of life and overall wellness of the patient is very important to the patient's ability to complete treatment, recover, and manage the side effects and potential complications.

Once a person is diagnosed with cancer, they often feel they have lost control of their life. The feeling of losing control takes an emotional and physical toll on the patient as well as their family. There is great value in the patient taking charge of even a small part of their care by paying attention to their nutrition, exercising, and exploring safe alternative treatments. It can provide an important feeling of control over a disease that often makes you feel out of control or that the disease is controlling you. This feeling of control can be a tremendous psychological lift for patients and their families as a means to cope and live their lives to the fullest extent.

IMPORTANCE OF OVERALL HEALTH

Let's talk about the importance of nutrition. Think of the body as a car. If your car has little gas, is fifteen years old, has 150,000 miles on the odometer, and has not had the oil changed in two years, driving anywhere may be a risk. You might be okay if you drive two miles to church, but if you attempt to drive across the country, it could be quite a challenge and probably a very bad idea.

Cancer is like a cross-country road trip. Your body is the car. If you smoke, are a hundred pounds overweight, eat refined sugar and processed foods, and your only exercise is getting off the couch, then your trip to fight your cancer is going to be very challenging.

The better functioning the car, the better running the engine, the better care you take of the vehicle, the better that car will do on the road trip. The same is true of your body—if you take care of your body with good nutrition, a good night's rest, and exercise, you'll have fewer treatment interruptions, less stress and anxiety, be better able to handle the side effects, and be much more likely to reach your destination through cancer treatment.

DIET

I'm a big believer in food as medicine, and while paying attention to your diet will not cure your GBM or HGG, it can go a long way toward making that journey easier on your body with fewer complications and side effects so you can still enjoy your life. A diet full of fruits and vegetables, healthy fats, lean proteins, and whole grains will put your body in a good place for the treatment ahead. A consult with a clinical dietician or nutritionist early in your care is highly recommended. Many comprehensive cancer centers provide these services, and I know of a few that actually have their own cooking and nutrition classes just for cancer patients.

You can also find several resources online. Here are a few:

www.oncologynutrition.org
has a section called "Eat Right to Fight Cancer."

www.thecancercoach.org
does free consultations and meal plans.

www.cancercare.org is very useful.

www.accc-cancer.org
Association of Community Cancer Centers has
a cancer nutrition resources section.

At the minimum, your doctor will recommend a balanced healthy diet, one that reflects whole foods and moderation. Remember, it's important to take good care of the "car" you're driving on the journey.

GENERAL DIETARY PRINCIPLES

A GBM patient needs a balanced diet, plenty of water, and basic nutrients for energy and healing. For any patient battling a chronic illness, we know that tight blood glucose control results in better recovery from illness and less severe illness. This is especially true if you are already diabetic. High blood glucose is associated with increased inflammation in the body and lower immune system function. Avoidance of foods high in refined or added sugar, such as soda, juices, candy, and doughnuts, is recommended. Increasing the number of whole grains, whole fruits, and vegetables will provide slowly digested sugars that will not cause harmful high spikes in blood sugar levels. Most GBM and HGG patients are frequently cycling on and off steroids, which will make control of blood sugar difficult. Using steroids only when necessary is important to avoid long-term side effects such as poor blood sugar control.

There are several foods that have anti-inflammatory properties that may be beneficial in reducing body-wide inflammation. Many of these foods are colorful fruits and vegetables that naturally contain plant-based chemicals that reduce inflammation. Additionally, poorly controlled glucose and most animal-based foods are associated with increased inflammation in the body. Reducing systemic inflammation through diet may reduce the patient's reliance on steroids and help avoid steroid-related side effects.

In addition to what we've already discussed, a balanced, well-structured diet that boosts the immune system, reduces systemic inflammation, keeps blood sugar levels low, and provides adequate protein will improve wound healing after surgery and decrease the risk of surgical infections and opportunistic infections related to steroid use.

KETOGENIC DIET

A ketogenic diet is a frequently discussed diet for cancer patients of all kinds, but it has been of particular interest in GBM, HGG, and other types of brain cancer.

Let's go through a quick introduction as to what the ketogenic diet is and what a ketone is. The ketogenic diet focuses on fats and proteins as the primary source of calories, with very little carbohydrates (sugar). Your body primarily wants to metabolize sugars as its energy source. If the body's supply of sugar (glucose and glycogen) is depleted, then your body will switch to protein and fat for energy.

When fat is metabolized, it produces a molecule called a ketone, which the body can also use for energy. Your level of ketones can be monitored in the blood or urine to determine if your body has gone into "ketosis," defined as a state where your body is depleted of glucose and has switched to fat and protein metabolism for energy. For *noncancer* patients, this can be used as a weight-loss diet.

Your brain loves to use ketones as an energy source, but your GBM/HGG hates ketones and is only interested in glucose (sugar) for energy. So, the theory is that if I put a GBM/HGG patient into ketosis through an ultra-low-sugar diet, then I am starving the tumor of its primary energy source (sugar), thus making it hard for the tumor to grow and thrive.

Sounds great, doesn't it? Of course, there's always a catch. Several useful studies have been done in animal models of GBM/HGG that demonstrated a benefit with the ketogenic diet. Unfortunately, there has not been a large enough study done in human GBM/HGG patients to convince the scientific community that the ketogenic diet increases survival or delays tumor progression. Several small studies have been done demonstrating the diet to be well tolerated and safe for GBM and HGG patients, but it has not shown to be effective in reducing the size of the GBM or HGG. Larger and more comprehensive studies are planned.

One obstacle to a large scientific study involving ketogenic diet and GBM/HGG is patient compliance. A ketogenic diet properly monitored for ketosis is difficult to adhere to and is a lot of work for the patient. Additionally, many GBM and HGG patients have the attitude that if this ultrastrict diet isn't a cure, then they prefer to eat the foods they truly enjoy.

ATTITUDE

The mind-body connection is a well-established belief that physical illness is linked to emotional and psychological health and biological factors. Our mind communicates with our body. How do we know that mood and attitude will influence our physical well-being? Good examples of this are how we respond to sadness, embarrassment, or nervousness—when we are sad, we cry; when we are embarrassed, we blush; and when we are nervous, we get "butterflies." Other examples of this connection include the effect of stress on blood pressure and the association between chronic pain and depression. Poorly controlled psychological stress can lead to high blood pressure, anxiety, worry, depression, fatigue, sleep disorders, and constipation or diarrhea, and can also manifest itself as chronic back, neck, or headache pain.

Repeated exposure to stress can make you ill. Treatment of stress, depression, and severe anxiety will often improve the symptoms. The body makes chemicals—norepinephrine, serotonin, endorphins—that boost our mood and fight against stress. Treatment can be as simple as trying different stress management techniques such as meditation, relaxation practices such as mindfulness or yoga, biofeedback, and exercise such as walking; spending time talking with people who care about you; writing a journal; or having massage therapies. If the anxiety or depression is severe, your treatment team may recommend that you see a mental health professional to determine whether medications are necessary.

A healthy attitude will help you on this journey. A positive attitude will not cure GBM and HGG, but when a patient is having trouble coping or is depressed, anxious, or very stressed, they will have more trouble tolerating medication, dealing with side effects, overcoming disabilities, and recovering from treatments. If a patient's mental health issues progress to the point that they give up and lose the will to live, a rapid decline in their health usually follows soon after.

TAKEAWAYS:

- There are no scientifically proven holistic or alternative treatments for GBM and HGG. However, the importance of sound nutrition, optimal overall health, and a positive mental attitude cannot be overstressed as you move through your treatments and care.

- Medical training is focused on treatments that have been scientifically evaluated for their effectiveness and safety. As a result, the medical community can sometimes have difficulty embracing treatments and care that has not been rigorously and scientifically evaluated.

- There is no diet that has been proven to be more beneficial to GBM and HGG patients. Balanced nutrition composed of nonprocessed whole foods will likely help the patient minimize the side effects of treatment and recover more quickly.

CHAPTER 12

FINANCIAL CONSIDERATIONS OF GBM

● ●

> Will my insurance company pay for the treatments?
>
> How can my doctor or cancer center help with my financial challenges?

Kevin's job as a welder included membership in a trade union. As part of his employment and union benefits, Kevin had very complete medical coverage, and outside of their normal deductibles, Kevin and his wife had few out-of-pocket expenses.

No single treatment, test, or hospital stay cost them any money once their deductible was paid. They did fly at their own expense to Phoenix, Arizona, to meet with specialists for a second opinion a couple of times.

In fact, Kevin actually made money during his treatment through a part of his union benefits he never knew he had. Kevin had what is called a "cancer rider." He contributed a small amount of each paycheck for this policy. Once he was diagnosed with cancer, this policy paid him directly a certain amount of money for every day in the hospital, every MRI, every emergency room visit. After several months of care, he had saved thousands of unexpected dollars, which he and his wife were saving for their children's college expenses!

HEALTHCARE IS EXPENSIVE, AND CANCER CARE IS SOME OF THE COSTLIEST.

Healthcare is expensive, and cancer care is some of the costliest. Ideally, it is best to be sure you understand what your health insurance policy covers before anyone gets ill, but in reality, many people do not pay attention to the details of their policy until they, or a family member, become ill or injured. As the cost of healthcare continues to increase, many hospitals have employed financial counselors or representatives who can explain your policy coverage to you.

TYPES OF MEDICAL COVERAGE

Discussed below are various forms of medical coverage that may be available to you.

MEDICARE

Age is the most frequent risk factor for cancer, and thus many patients who need cancer care are Medicare beneficiaries. Medicare is a federal program that persons over the age of sixty-five are eligible for. This is health insurance that is funded by the US government and US taxpayers. Medicare is divided into Medicare A and Medicare B. Medicare part A covers expenses billed during a hospitalization. This would include expenses such as room and board while in the hospital along with all testing, medications, imaging, and surgical services. There is usually a deductible that the patient is responsible for as part of Medicare A. Medicare part B covers expenses billed as part of outpatient care. As long as the doctor accepts Medicare, the Medicare part B coverage will take care of 80 percent of what your doctor bills for approved cancer treatments, office visits, and testing related to your cancer diagnosis as an outpatient. The patient will be responsible for 20 percent of the billed amount unless they purchase a Medicare Supplemental Plan that covers the other 20 percent.

Basic Medicare part B may not cover prescription drugs, including chemotherapy. Medicare patients, and especially cancer patients, should consider purchasing some sort of prescription drug coverage, usually in the form of a Medicare part D plan or as part of a Medicare Advantage plan.

The American Cancer Society Cancer Action Network has a free publication on their website that is informative for patients who need to understand health insurance and cancer care: www.fightcancer.org/sites/default/files/Costs%20of%20Cancer%20-%20Final%20Web.pdf.

MEDICAID AND NO MEDICAL INSURANCE

Persons without health insurance of any kind will be responsible for all of their treatment costs. Uninsured patients may be able to negotiate discounts with providers and/or hospitals. Some hospitals have patient assistance or "charity care" programs, and they may be able to enroll the patient in pharmaceutical company drug discount programs to help reduce their costs.

Patients who do not have insurance may be eligible for state-sponsored insurance for low-income households, often referred to as *Medicaid*. Patients with Medicaid may find that their options for where, who, and how their cancer is treated are more limited. Medicaid programs vary from state to state. The rules, regulations, and extent of coverage may be different in California compared to Florida. Who is covered, what is covered, and how much your out-of-pocket cost will be will also vary. The patient will also need to *qualify* for Medicaid benefits based on their financial situation. If you make too much money, you may not qualify.

Another important reality about Medicaid is that some medical facilities and doctors may not take Medicaid as payment or may limit the number of Medicaid patients they can care for.

PRIVATE OR EMPLOYER MEDICAL INSURANCE

For patients with private or employer-sponsored insurance, the type of health insurance and the benefit structure are the most important components in determining the costs for patients. To understand what your personal financial responsibility will be for any care you receive, become familiar with the language in your policy that describes the monthly premium, the deductible, copayment or copay, co-insurance, out-of-pocket maximum or cap terminology, and *which providers and hospitals are considered to be "in network."* Should you choose to go to a provider or a hospital that is not included "in network" of your health insurance payer, it will be important to understand what the "out-of-network" limitations and benefits include. Copays and deductibles may be higher when choosing out-of-network care. Out-of-network care may also require additional permission or authorization from the insurer.

WHAT DOES A DEDUCTIBLE MEAN?

Often, cancer care requires inpatient care, outpatient doctor appointments, surgery, radiation, expensive medications, imaging studies, and the list goes on and on. Let's look at an example with an insurance plan that has a $1,000 a year deductible limit: A person has a seizure and is taken to the local emergency room. The ER doctor gives him or her medication to treat the seizure and orders a CT scan of the head and then an MRI to look for a cause for the seizure. By this time, after four hours in the ER and all the testing and care that has occurred, the cost incurred will have met the $1,000 deductible for the year. This means that at some point the patient owes $1,000 for these medical services. But any other medical care needed that year should be covered by the insurance company if it is included as a covered benefit under the policy.

RETURNING TO WORK AND DISABILITY BENEFITS

As discussed in earlier chapters, the diagnosis of GBM or HGG may result in permanent or temporary, physical, or cognitive disability that may make working impossible. Additionally, the diagnosis of GBM or HGG may also cause the patient to rethink their priorities in life, and returning to work may not be high on the list compared to spending time with family and loved ones. Should the need arise, applying for Social Security Disability or taking advantage of a long-term disability insurance policy may provide needed income if the patient with GBM or HGG is no longer able to work.

Even if you could physically still work, the diagnosis of GBM/HGG all by itself very often will qualify a patient for a long-term disability benefit. If you are applying for Social Security Disability, an attorney who specializes in disability claims can be very helpful and can result in faster approval of benefits.

For other patients, returning to work may provide a much-needed distraction from their diagnosis and provide a feeling of stability and an opportunity for socialization. Some people really like their job and prefer to continue to work. But for some GBM/HGG patients, returning to work may not be for the best, and it's important to realize that applying for disability support is an option.

OTHER INSURANCE BENEFITS

Another benefit that may be available is an insurance policy called a "cancer policy" or "critical illness policy." These are insurance riders and are usually offered through an employer. These policy riders cover expenses associated with the diagnosis of cancer or a severe illness that requires intensive/critical care. These policies are often very reasonably priced, and some people purchase these policies years before and forget they exist.

Cancer or critical illness policies may provide payment *on top* of your normal medical insurance. For example, a GBM/HGG patient requires an MRI every three months. *Their medical insurance will pay the MRI facility for the MRI. If they have a cancer policy, that policy may pay $800 directly to the patient. Here's another example: After surgery, a GBM patient may spend two days in the intensive care unit (ICU). Their medical insurance will pay the hospital for their days in the ICU. If they have a critical illness policy, that policy may pay $1,000 directly to the patient for each day in the ICU. Again, this is money* in addition to their medical insurance paying the bills.

The diagnosis of GBM or HGG is enough stress and worry in the life of any patient and their family. Anything that can reduce the added stress of money and finances should be taken advantage of without guilt or remorse. Many major hospital centers and cancer centers provide financial counseling to patients and families and can be very helpful sorting through the options that may be available. If not, you can contact the insurance company, and they can explain what is covered and not covered in your policy.

TAKEAWAYS:

- Each patient's healthcare coverage is different regarding cancer care. It is important to become familiar with your coverage.

- Insurance coverage is complicated, but most hospitals and cancer centers provide financial counseling and assistance.

- Even if you have no insurance at the beginning of your diagnosis, there are options and programs to help you make sure your costs are met.

CHAPTER 13

OTHER CARE PATHS TO PURSUE OR CONSIDER

How can I enroll in an experimental trial?

What steps need to be taken to prepare my family for the diagnosis of GBM?

When Kevin's GBM recurred, I had several talks with Kevin and his wife about what this recurrence meant and what options were available. Kevin had his second surgery to remove his recurrent GBM, and we placed Gliadel wafers into the surgical site. Once the wound healed, Kevin and his wife also decided to start the Optune system.

About four months later, I saw Kevin in the office for his regular visit. He was losing weight, moving slower, and in general seemed detached and not very animated in our discussion. He also started to develop a very subtle weakness in his right arm, and his right leg was lagging behind when he walked.

When I looked at Kevin's MRI, my heart sank. Kevin's tumor had recurred for a third time, but this time it was in an entirely new location, far from his original tumor and in a deep place that surgery couldn't reach. Additionally, the MRI showed the tumor had become "multicentric," meaning that instead of one tumor, the MRI showed several separate clusters of tumors—a very bad sign.

I gave the news to Kevin and his wife, and of course they were disappointed. I explained that at this point another surgery would not be an option and that Kevin had essentially exhausted all the standard available treatments for GBM. Their only option at this point for further treatment was if Kevin could be accepted to an experimental clinical trial.

Kevin and Julie went home to consider their options and decided that they were not interested in seeking any further treatment, but they wanted to continue clinic visits to follow Kevin's condition.

At the beginning of this book, the lack of a cure for GBM and HGG was mentioned. GBM and HGG are treatable, but only in very rare instances are they curable. Current treatments focus on reducing the amount of tumor, reducing symptoms, and delaying new or regrowth of tumor.

THE WORSE THE CONDITION OF THE PATIENT, THE FEWER TREATMENT OPTIONS WILL BE AVAILABLE.

Families and patients may decide to not continue treatment for various reasons. Some of the most common scenarios seen include the following:

- One possible situation concerns the overall health or medical condition of the patient. Most treatments, surgical or chemotherapeutic, depend on the patient being in good enough condition to tolerate the treatment. The worse the condition of the patient, the fewer treatment options will be available.

If the patient's overall condition and level of function are poor, the patient may not be able to tolerate whatever treatment remains available.

- Another situation patients may find themselves in is simply running out of treatment options. If the patient has gone through all the conventional treatments of radiation, multiple surgeries, first-, second-, even third-line chemotherapy and been evaluated and screened for experimental treatments, there may be nothing left for your treatment team to offer.

- Additionally, like Kevin and Julie, the patient and their family may decide to just stop treatments. Choosing to do nothing is always an option, especially when dealing with an incurable disease. Some patients will choose to have no treatments at all. They prefer to enjoy their remaining time without the risks and side effects associated with the treatments. It is the doctor's job to be sure that the patient is mentally competent to make such a decision and to be sure they understand the consequences of that decision.

EXPERIMENTAL TRIALS

Numerous clinical trials for the treatment of GBM and HGG are being conducted all over the country by hundreds of dedicated researchers, universities, and biomedical/pharmaceutical companies. The sheer scope and number of trials make it difficult for any individual doctor to monitor and understand the details of them all. Most doctors involved in GBM and HGG treatment will be familiar and have access to enroll patients in a few, but certainly not all, available clinical trials.

Trials are being done exploring the use of vaccines, immunotherapy, radiation and chemotherapy combinations, different combinations of new chemotherapy, and new and innovative surgical technologies as well as the analysis of genetic and molecular markers to better target tumors.

Finding and understanding clinical trials can be an overwhelming and daunting task for your treatment team, never mind a patient and their family. Fortunately, several organizations have developed tools to help families and their treatment teams find and understand clinical trials that may be available.

NATIONAL BRAIN TUMOR SOCIETY, TRIALS.BRAINTUMOR.ORG

BRAIN TUMOR FOUNDATION, BRAINTUMORFOUNDATION.ORG

UNIVERSITY OF PENNSYLVANIA TRIAL MATCHING AND REFERRAL SERVICE, ONCOLINK.ORG

The National Brain Tumor Society has a very easy-to-use tool to find clinical trials and link you to a trial point of contact. Go to Trials.braintumor.org for more information. The Brain Tumor Foundation (BTF), Braintumorfoundation.org, website has a very comprehensive list of clinical trial resources under the "Knowledge is Power" tab. The University of Pennsylvania provides the Trial Matching and Referral Service (Oncolink.org). Most of these clinical trial resources will provide a questionnaire that asks for details specific about your GBM, how you've been treated, how well you responded to the treatment, what genetic or molecular markers your tumor has, and then matches you to clinical trials within a certain distance. You may need a member of your treatment team to help you fill out this questionnaire but it only takes a few minutes. I have found these tools very useful and often utilize them when searching for clinical trials for my own patients.

It is important to understand that just because you want to be involved in an experimental clinical trial doesn't mean you will qualify or be accepted for that trial. Experimental trials are run under a strict set of specifications that are designed to answer very specific questions about the particular treatment that is being studied. If for whatever reason you don't fit into the specifications, then you won't be accepted into the trial. Age, sex, weight, other medical problems, genetic markers of your GBM, and other treatments you've had all may qualify or disqualify you from a trial. This can sometimes be frustrating and hard to understand for patients because they have often run out of standard treatments and may have trouble understanding why these rules are important.

I would recommend you talk to your treatment team about your interest in clinical trials. Members of your treatment team should be able to help guide you and help you sort through the clinical trials available in your area.

PLANNING

A life-threatening illness often compels patients and families to plan ahead for all likely circumstances. It is important for peace of mind for both the patient and the family. This is the time when many families will turn to a spiritual advisor, such as a chaplain or a minister, as well as to a financial or legal advisor. While no patient or family wants to discuss end-of-life planning, it would be wise for families to discuss important legal and financial issues associated with a terminal illness as soon as there is some understanding of the patient's prognosis. This is not a book about financial planning and legal advice, but basic considerations such as making a will, the management of debts and assets, and sharing the locations, account numbers and passwords for financial-related accounts should be well thought out in advance.

ADVANCED DIRECTIVES

Regardless of where the patient is in their diagnosis and treatment journey, the patient should talk to their family and write down their wishes. There are specific documents or forms available from all hospitals and from lawyers. In general, there are three types of documents you should be familiar with to help communicate your wishes. These documents may be called a *healthcare proxy*, an *advanced directive*, a *living will*, or a *power of attorney*.

Each of these documents accomplishes a different goal, and they can be confusing at times. According to the website of the Heritage Law Center (www.maheritagelawcenter.com), a *healthcare proxy or medical power of attorney* allows you to choose a person, "known as an *agent or proxy*, to legally make healthcare decisions for you" when you are unable to do so. What does that mean? It means that if I appoint my brother as my healthcare proxy or medical power of attorney, he is allowed to make any decision regarding my medical care if I can't. For example, if I need surgery, my brother is empowered to give permission. If the doctors want to take me off a ventilator because all hope is lost, my brother has to say it's okay.

An *advanced directive,* also known as a *living will,* "expresses your wishes as to how your agent should proceed in certain specific circumstances" when the patient cannot do so themselves. If I fill out and sign an advanced directive, then I have spelled out specific medical situations and how I want to be treated in those situations. For example, my advanced directive may say that if my heart stops and I stop breathing, then I do not want to be put on a ventilator or have my heart restarted with medication and CPR. If I suffer a stroke or a very bad brain injury, my advanced directive may say that I don't want treatment if it means I will live in a nursing home or be dependent on others for my routine care. An advanced directive tells my medical team and family what I would want done in certain situations.

A power of attorney (POA) is a legal document that authorizes another person to act on your behalf. A POA is usually limited to business, legal, and financial matters for the time when the patient is unavailable or not capable of taking those actions. For example, my wife is my POA, which allows her to draw on my bank accounts, access my money, and pay my bills if I cannot. A POA is *not* a document that appoints a person to make medical decisions unless it specifically states that they are empowered to make decisions regarding medical care.

Your POA and healthcare proxy can be the same person. It is also important to understand that if the patient does *not* have a healthcare proxy, it's okay. The doctors will work with the patient's next of kin to make decisions.

CHANGING CONDITIONS

As the patient's condition changes, the doctors will make sure the patient's decline isn't due to a reversible and treatable problem. Sometimes a GBM/HGG patient's condition may change or worsen for reasons not related to tumor progression or recurrence. A patient may worsen due to an increase in brain swelling that can be treated with steroids, a urinary tract infection that can be treated with antibiotics, and seizures that can be treated with antiseizure medications. The patient or family should contact the treatment team with any new or worsening symptoms. Your team may recommend an MRI or testing to determine the cause of the change. But there will be a time when the only reason for the decline is the progression of the GBM/HGG.

As the GBM/HGG progresses, most patients will not experience pain. They may become confined to bed as the result of weakness or the loss of the ability to walk. They may spend more time sleeping. They may become confused and have difficulty thinking. This change occurs gradually, usually over the course of several weeks, until the patient slips into an unconscious state and does not awaken. When it becomes impossible for the family to provide all the care that the patient will need at home, palliative and hospice care may be considered. Palliative and hospice care is a special field of medicine whose focus is to improve the quality of life and reduce suffering for patients with serious illness. Some hospitals will have palliative care or hospice inpatient beds, but palliative and hospice professionals can also provide home care to ensure that the patient and the family are supported and comfortable.

TAKEAWAYS:

- There are dozens of experimental trials being conducted at any given time. Not all patients will qualify for trials. The major brain tumor research organizations provide tools to help the patient find an appropriate trial.

- For the sake of the patient and the surviving family, it is important to plan for the financial and emotional issues associated with the diagnosis of GBM.

CONCLUDING THOUGHTS

. . . .

The diagnosis of GBM or HGG alters the course of life for the patient, their friends, and their family. In the beginning, processing and coping with a new diagnosis of GBM or HGG is full of emotional ups and downs. The patient may be hopeful one day, scared the next day, and later angry. One day your life is familiar, predictable, and stable. Then suddenly you're faced with new people and places and fears. Trying to understand unfamiliar and strange medical language. Making important decisions about your care with difficult-to-understand information. Putting your life and trust in a process that may initially look terrifying and complicated. Learning to put your life and faith in the hands of people you don't know, and learning to trust that their only concern is what is best for you and that they desperately want to offer you comfort, help, and reassurance.

Here are a few important points to remember that I want to leave the patient and their families and friends with:

1. Remember, the medical professionals who are taking care of you (your physicians, nurses, technicians, etc.) are all very smart, highly educated, and well trained. The people who

work in cancer centers dedicated their professional careers to helping cancer patients like you. I encourage you to have faith in these dedicated professionals. They are focused on gaining your trust, providing the best services available, and working toward maximizing your treatment while minimizing your discomfort.

2. Medicine is not a perfect science. Your treatment team is going to recommend the best treatments and care for you based on their experience and what the highest-quality medical data demonstrates.

3. This journey is a lot easier surrounded by the ones you love and people who care about you.

4. *Don't. Lose. Hope.* In the fifteen years I have been involved in brain tumor research and treatment, there have been at least five major additions and changes to the standard of treatment for GBM and HGG. That is more progress in fifteen years than in the previous fifty! Medicine's understanding of GBM and HGG increases every year. Thousands of people have dedicated their lives to finding better treatments and a cure. Millions, if not billions, of dollars are being spent toward a cure and treatments.

I hope this book provides readers with a resource they can use throughout their journey. I hope this book arms them with the knowledge to make informed decisions so they may take some measure of control during this roller coaster ride and be an active, informed, and positive contributor to their treatment. This book is designed to provide patients and families a starting point to understand what to expect on this journey and a reference point they can always return to when the road changes and new challenges arise.

Please feel free to use my website, www.drthomasgruber.com, as a source for the latest updates on treatments and innovations in the treatment of GBM, HGG, and a variety of other neurologic conditions. I welcome you to visit it and look at the information provided there whenever you are looking for the most recent news on GBM and HGG.

ABOUT THE AUTHORS

Dr. Thomas Gruber is a Board Certified Neurosurgeon whose primary focus is cancer treatment of the brain, spine and nervous system. After serving in the US Army, he graduated from medical school and completed his residency in neurosurgery at the University of Buffalo, Buffalo, New York. Dr. Gruber trained in neuro-oncology and brain tumor treatments at Roswell Park Cancer Center in Buffalo, New York. While at Roswell Park Cancer Center, he also conducted brain tumor research and was the author of numerous publications. He is currently Chief of Surgery at Baptist Health Hospital System in Western Kentucky, where he works with a team of cancer specialists at the Eckstein Regional Cancer Center to provide the most up-to-date treatments available for all tumors and cancer diagnoses affecting the brain, spine and nervous system.

Ms. Marcia Gruber-Page is a registered nurse with a diverse clinical and administrative healthcare background. Marcia has three master's degrees (adult oncology, epidemiology, and leadership) and has been active at the national level in the Oncology Nursing Society and the

Society for Gastroenterology Nurses & Associates, Inc. Marcia is a reviewer for the *Clinical Journal of Oncology Nursing* and a mentor for aspiring oncology nurse writers. She has forty-plus publications and has presented locally, regionally, and nationally on topics such as patient care, nursing, quality, and building outpatient cancer facilities. Marcia has held oncology administrator positions at two NCI Cancer Centers—Roswell Park Cancer Institute and MD Anderson Cancer Center—and was the Vice President for Oncology for the Dignity Health Cancer Institute at St. Joseph's Hospital and Medical Center in Phoenix, Arizona. Marcia is currently the System Vice President for Oncology for the CommonSpirit Health Oncology Clinical Institute. Marcia leads the CSH Oncology Clinical Institute with her Physician Dyad partner, and they are responsible for leading and developing strategies for the Oncology Clinical Institute and Service Line. She provides leadership across the continuum, leads the adoption of clinical quality standards and performance improvement initiatives to increase quality, improve outcomes, eliminate unnecessary variation, and enhance care coordination for the fifty-plus oncology programs across the twenty-one states served by CommonSpirit Health.

CONTACT US

WWW.DRTHOMASGRUBER.COM

NOTES

Printed in the USA
CPSIA information can be obtained
at www.ICGtesting.com
JSHW081706170624
64967JS00004B/193